ANNE HOOPER'S
ULTIMATE
SEX
POSITIONS

OVER 100 POSITIONS
FOR MAXIMUM EROTIC
PLEASURE

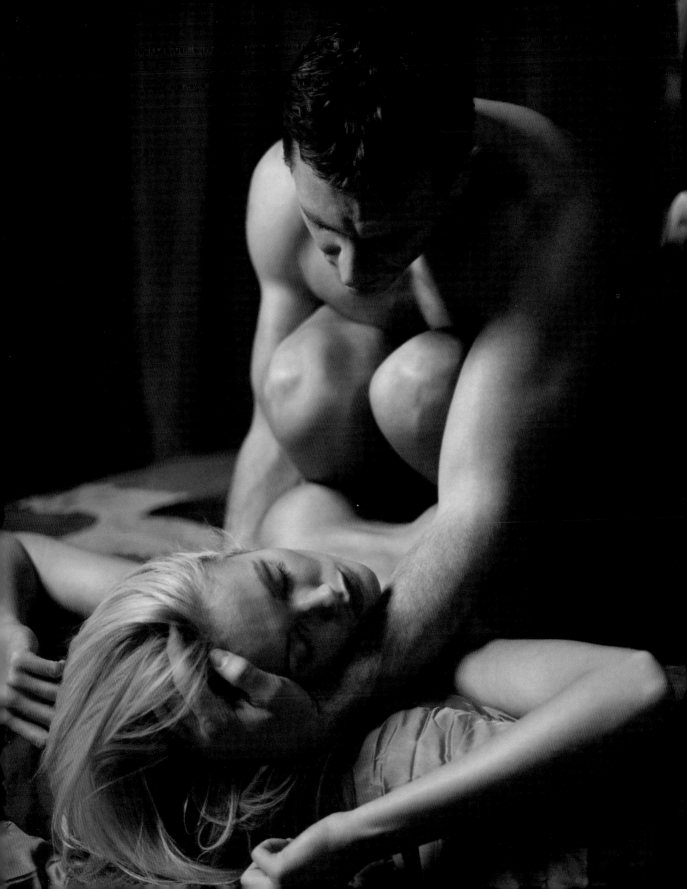

ANNE HOOPER'S
ULTIMATE
SEX
POSITIONS

OVER 100 POSITIONS
FOR MAXIMUM EROTIC
PLEASURE

LONDON, NEW YORK, MUNICH,
MELBOURNE, and DELHI

Editor Daniel Mills
Art Editor Katherine Raj
Executive Managing Editor Adèle Hayward
Managing Art Editor Kat Mead
Production Editor Kelly Salih
Senior Production Editor Jenny Woodcock
Creative Technical Support Sonia Charbonnier
Production Controller Mandy Inness
Art Director Peter Luff
Publisher Stephanie Jackson
US Editor Chuck Wills

PRODUCED FOR DK BY
Louise Frances (**Editor**) And Collette Sadler (**Designer**).
First American Edition, 2009

Published in the United States by
DK Publishing
375 Hudson Street
New York, New York 10014

09 10 11 12   10 9 8 7 6 5 4 3 2 1

175527—December 2009

Published in Great Britain by Dorling Kindersley Limited.

A CIP catalog record for this book
is available from the Library of Congress.

ISBN 978-0-7566-5569-3

Color reproduction by MDP, UK
Printed in Singapore by Star Standard

See our complete catalog at
www.dk.com

Previously published in Kama Sutra for 21st Century Lovers, Sex Play, Sexopedia, XXX Sex... Tonight!

DK books are available at special discounts when purchased in bulk for sales promotions, premiums,
fund-raising, or educational use. For details, contact: DK Publishing Special Markets,
375 Hudson Street, New York, New York 10014 or SpecialSales@dk.com.

Contents

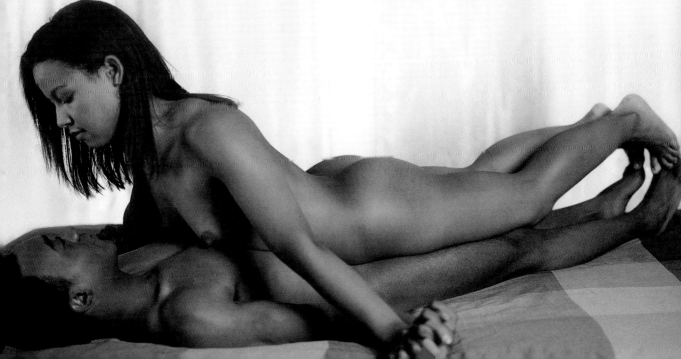

Introduction

Sex can be the greatest source of pleasure and happiness in our lives—it can boost our personal sense of well-being and health, and it also fosters precious feelings of intimacy with a partner. I believe that most lovers want to understand more about their partner's psyche, and be able to connect with them on much deeper levels. Nowhere is the need for this understanding more apparent than in the bedroom.

Sexual Variety

If good sex is important, nothing kills good sex quicker than boredom. However much you adore your partner, if you have made love in the same way, in the same bed, in the same room for years, things just aren't as erotic as they used to be. Change only one item in that pattern, and sex takes on a new lease of life.

The secret is to keep an open mind, and be unafraid to make some slightly different moves. To help you to keep your own relationship vibrant, I have compiled a collection of orgasm-enhancing sexual techniques and positions for all kinds of pleasure, intimacy, and fun.

Erotic Embraces

The cornerstone of any relationship is intimacy, and the first chapter highlights the importance of closeness, with positions devoted to comfort and romance. Cleansing the body, relaxing the mind, dimming the lights, and playing sensual music all figure in the love plan. I would suggest the addition of a glass or two to drink, a light meal, the gift of playful massage, and oceans of time.

In this chapter, I've also explored the world of erotic treats—if you've ever wondered how to give a sexual massage, or stimulate your lover's body using just your teeth, this is the place to find out.

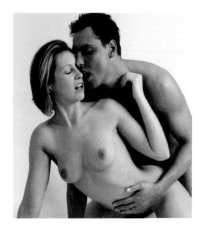 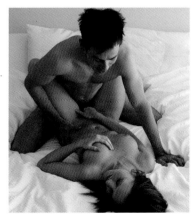 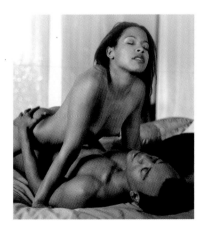

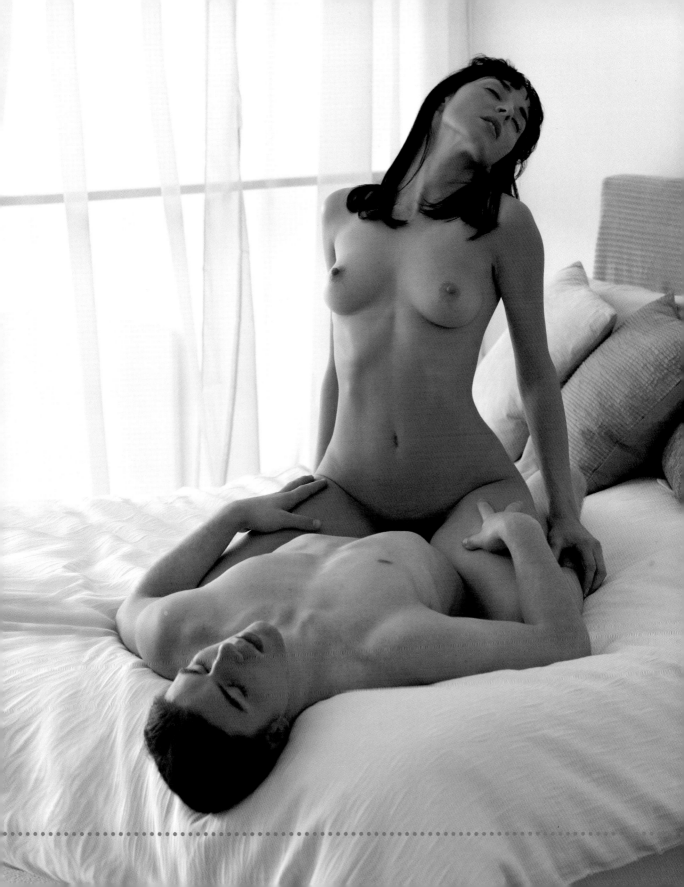

Maximum Sensation

The positions in this chapter aim to give maximum stimulation to both partners, to help both of you to experience intense pleasure. At its best, sexual intercourse can resemble a wonderful series of flowing movements. There are rare but blissful moments where physical sensation is so heightened that every action, movement, and stroke feels as though you are floating. This is the result of every nerve cell in the body being so stimulated that every single action feels sensational. Chapter 2 also covers stimulation you can offer your partner, with techniques for manual and oral sex.

Acrobatic Ecstasy

This chapter is devoted to more adventurous positions requiring a degree of suppleness, and a desire to experiment. Many of the most demanding come from ancient sex manuals such as the *Kama Sutra*, but I have tried to keep a modern perspective on these age-old positions. This sometimes includes a certain irreverence on my part when, for example, I mention that a particular sexual position can be enjoyed only by the most supple of acrobats. The humor inherent in many of the most exotic descriptions of sex positions is irresistible. You might find that some of them may not do a lot for your orgasms, but you'll have fabulous fun performing them!

I've also included ideas to add excitement, such as taking sex out of the bedroom. Virtually any room can be an erotic venue, as long as you are assured of privacy, and after all, life is too short to make love only in bed. To add further variety, I've included a brief guide to tantric sex—a spiritual approach to lovemaking that aims to enrich the mind and soul, as well as provide sensual pleasure.

Sex Games and Adventures

Today sex is experienced not just as a private activity between two people, but also as a statement of lifestyle and fashion. Chapter 4 is intended to appeal to all loving couples who fancy moving onto the slightly more adventurous sides of love, but in a way that feels safe and unthreatening.

Sex games are a fantastic antidote to sexual boredom—they can turn ordinary lovemaking into something exciting and charged with sexual tension. Taking on different roles,

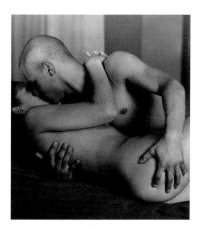
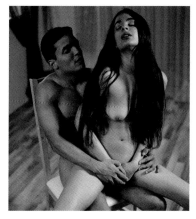
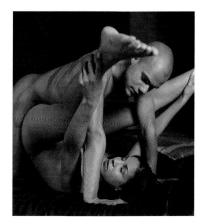

acting out erotic fantasies and using sexy props can really turn up the heat in your sex life. I've suggested a range of games, from unconventional positions to opportunities for fantasy and roleplay.

The final chapter will also help you become a sexpert when it comes to choosing and using erotic toys. Today, people are more open to the idea of experimentation in bed, and there is a constant demand for sexual novelty. More and more sex toys and DVDs are being sold, and the range is increasing all the time. The Internet has made sex toys easy to access and buy. Although women are buying many erotic novelties, every sex item bought by a woman also gets scrutinized by the man in her life. So, whether you are a man or a woman, it's useful to know your way around the world of pumps, rings, beads, dildos, and vibrators.

Intimate Trust

Old-fashioned concepts of trust and respect are vital ingredients for creating a sense of intimacy and spiritual peace between long-term partners, and many people possess a fragile self-confidence that is especially vulnerable during lovemaking. Inhibition in both partners is an obvious hindrance to intimate sex. So, too, is the fear that if you disclose sexual secrets to someone intimate you expose yourself somehow to their power or you negatively alter the relationship.

I believe that it's possible to replace fear with energy and enthusiasm to achieve a far deeper intimacy. Make sure your partner is aware of how much you love, trust, and admire them, and that they can trust you in turn. Then, make a resolution with your lover to throw away your inhibitions. Your sex life can blossom as a result. If you've never tried something before, don't worry about looking silly. Your only goals should be to explore, experiment, and—above all—to have fun.

I hope that, as well as learning skillful techniques, readers will be reminded of the fact that sex can be spiritually uplifting. If you believe this, I hope you will welcome the idea of using loving sex as a gateway to spirituality. Ultimately, I hope that you, the reader, will gain new insights into your own character and behavior, and be able to make amazing love to your adored partner.

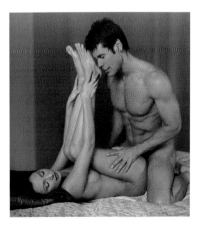 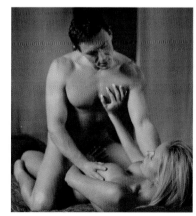 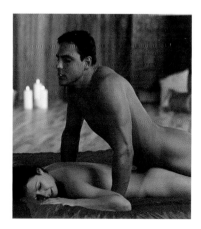

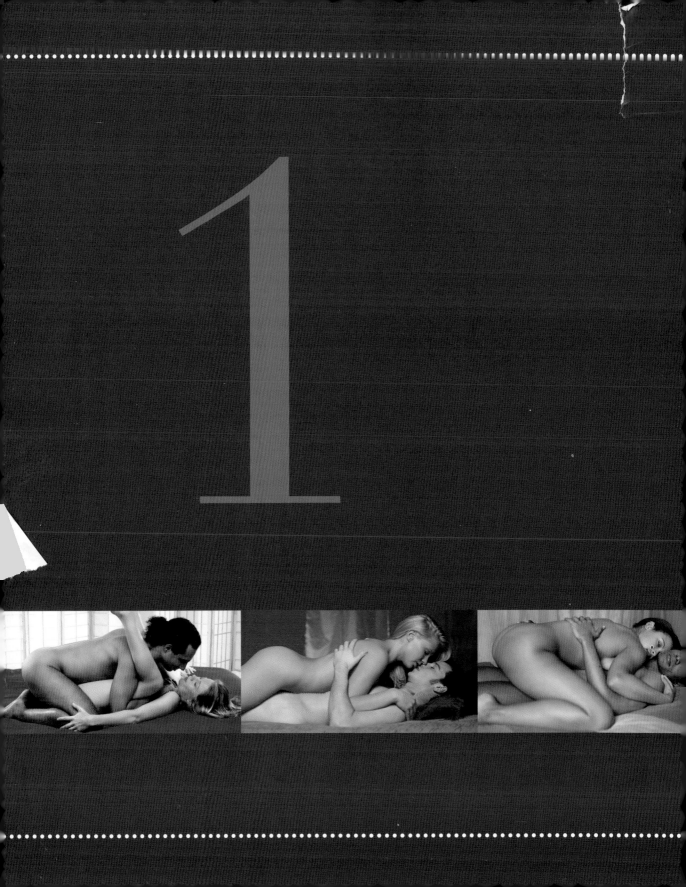

Erotic Embraces

Sex brings couples closer together both physically and emotionally. As well as forging a connection between bodies, the best lovemaking fosters a sense of intimacy and attachment. Even though we may no longer feel the same intense sexual buzz in a long-term relationship, intimate feelings act as a reminder of the special days at the beginning of a relationship, and help to bind us together.

Here you'll find plenty of positions where you can cuddle up tight with your lover. Rediscover the full body-to-body, feel-good intimacy of the missionary position in poses such as the Sexy Crush and Intimate Wraparound. Enjoy sliding in and out of each other's erotic embrace in the Lovers' Vine or Legs Entwined. Nuzzle up to your partner in Spoons or enjoy some cushioned loving in Sexy Embrace.

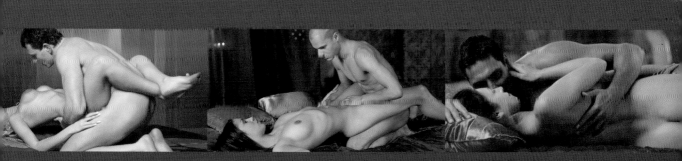

• MASSAGE STROKES FOR HIM

A woman can enhance her partner's sexual experience during lovemaking by gliding her hands smoothly from the top of his thighs over his bottom, and cupping his buttocks in her hands. These strokes may be experienced as a rush of sensation, especially if her movement is tantalizingly slow. Alternate light finger touch with deeper pressure using the palms of your hands. Keep your movements slow and sexy to send tingles of excitement all along his spine.

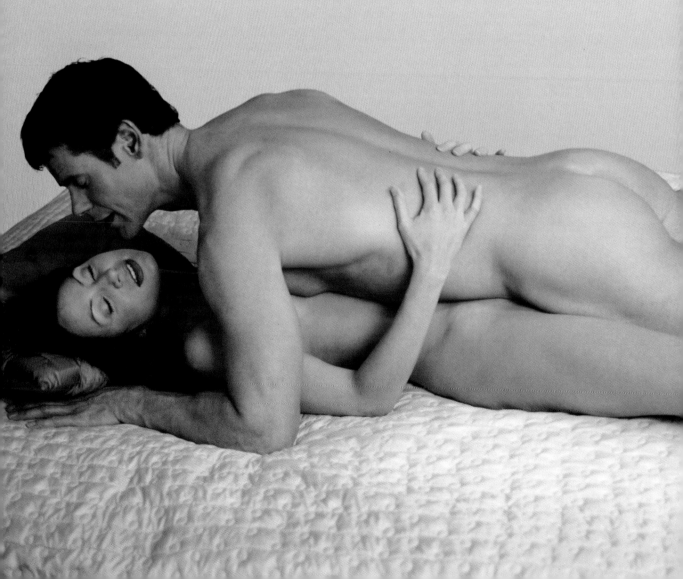

relaxed and intimate

Kiss each other to ecstasy in the classic missionary position

The missionary position offers full body-to-body contact, feels good, and is particularly comfortable for the woman. Lying face-to-face, the couple can experience the magic of skin against skin, with his entire body covering hers.

In the missionary position, the woman lies on her back while her partner lies on top of her, but supports his upper body weight on his forearms to begin thrusting. She opens her legs, and lays them out flat on the bed with her knees slightly bent. Then either partner can guide the penis into the vagina. The depth of penetration that is achieved in this position creates intensely pleasurable stimulation for both partners.

Men: the movement of sex will pull her labia rhythmically across her clitoris, and create a gentle, stimulating friction that is highly arousing. However, the missionary position does not necessarily bring a woman to climax, so spend some time stroking her clitoris before penetrating her.

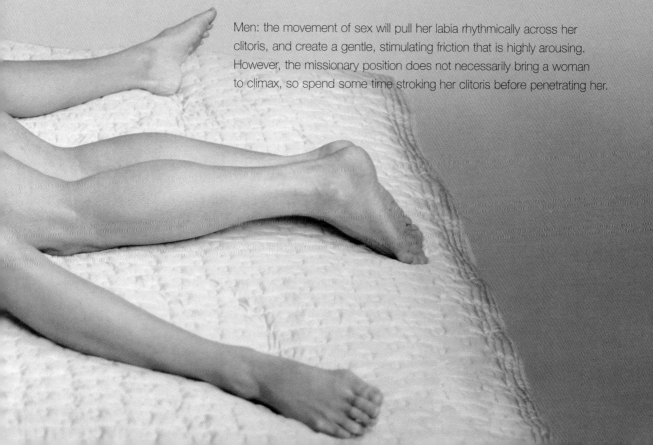

legs entwined

Enhance intimacy and treat your lover to a full-body embrace

Weaving and twining your arms and legs around each other is part of the intricate, unspoken choreography of love, and enables lovers to get close.

Full-body touch and friction inevitably triggers feelings of powerful sexual excitement. With legs and arms intertwined, this position encourages the couple to make love while clinging to each other in an intense,

passionate embrace. If the woman wraps her legs around her lover's body she can take a more active role by controlling the tempo and depth of his thrusts.

The man's gentle rocking movements build excitement, and friction between the couple, as she holds him tightly with her legs to gain the most physical pleasure from lovemaking. The tender intimacy of this position can arouse both of you, and enhance orgasm.

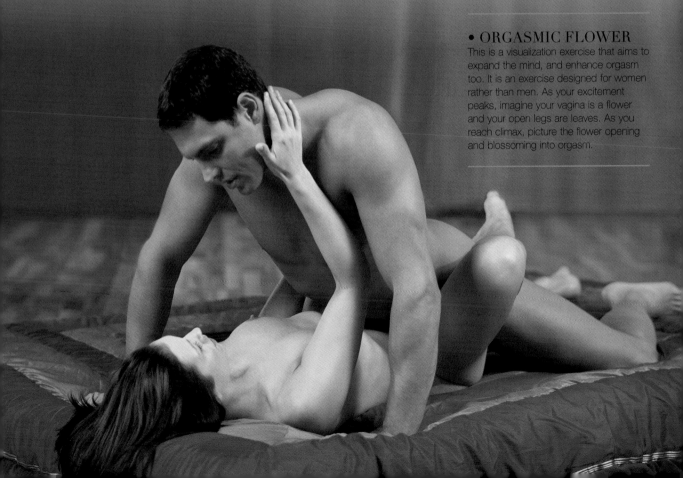

• ORGASMIC FLOWER
This is a visualization exercise that aims to expand the mind, and enhance orgasm too. It is an exercise designed for women rather than men. As your excitement peaks, imagine your vagina is a flower and your open legs are leaves. As you reach climax, picture the flower opening and blossoming into orgasm.

face to face

The missionary position is wonderfully diverse and changeable. Here, the couple takes a break from extreme closeness. The man raises himself up on his arms, while she tenderly strokes his buttocks.

In this position, the man can look down to watch himself thrusting in, and out of his lover. To get closer to him, she can raise her hips up high so that her pelvis presses against his. Putting a cushion beneath her buttocks will tilt her pelvis upward and allow for

deeper penetration. In return, the woman can show how eager she is for lovemaking by wrapping her arms and legs passionately around his body.

Men: during penetration, position her clitoris against the base of your penis. Rub softly side to side, and round and round, so that she is fully stimulated.

Women: the area between your man's anus and penis is full of nerve endings. Reach between his legs to cup and stroke his testicles gently from underneath.

• BREAST STROKES

Some women (but not all) have incredibly sensitive breasts and nipples. While your man is busy thrusting, touch yourself with firm strokes first, then repeat the touch with lighter strokes. Finally use your fingertips only. The stroking sensation will enhance your excitement during lovemaking, and that's good for both of you.

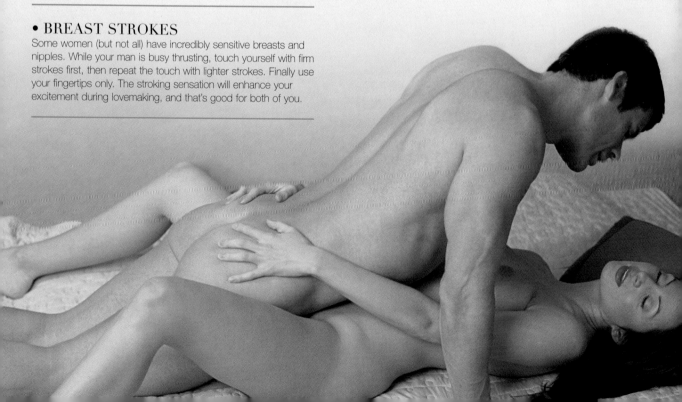

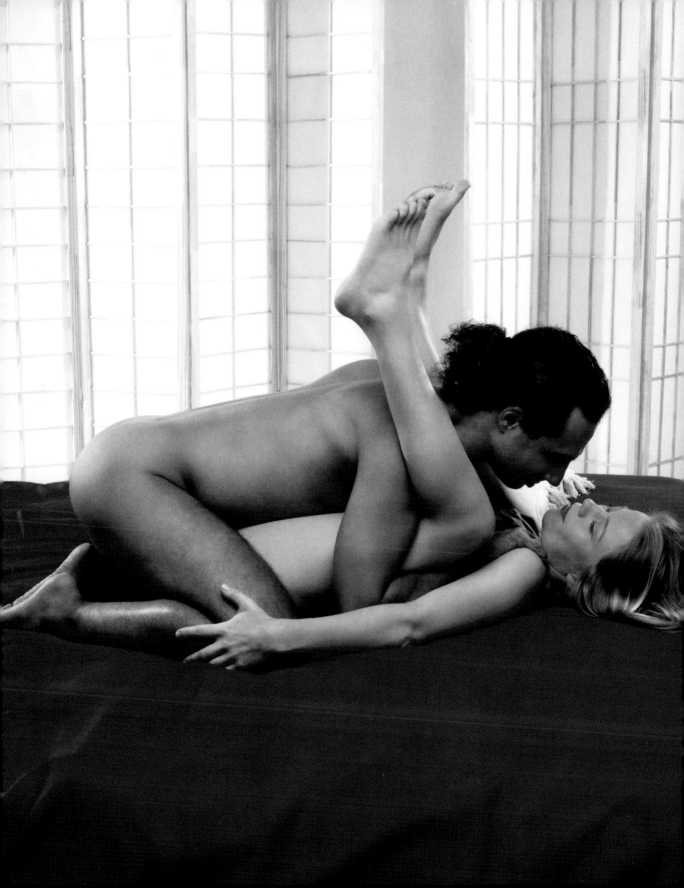

sexy crush

Many men and women are excited by the sensation of crushing, or being crushed by, their partner's body. There is an eroticism aroused by rough, tight body contact during sex.

In this variation of the missionary, the woman lies back and lifts her legs high so that the man finds it easy to penetrate her. He can thrust deep inside her body, to experience extreme sensations along his penis. Once inside her, he can relax, letting his weight down onto his elbows. This has the advantage that the couple's faces are close enough to allow passionate kissing.

However, if the man is considerably heavier than his partner, it may be necessary for him to lift himself up occasionally on his arms to avoid his full weight from bearing down on her. This will also change the angle of entry of his penis, and allow him to penetrate more deeply, giving her more clitoral stimulation.

The woman may feel vulnerable in this position, both literally and figuratively, as her legs are raised helplessly above her man's shoulders. A woman might suggest this position when she is deeply in love, and wants to show her feelings of trust and dependency.

Couples might even find that this pose awakens deeper sexual fantasies about submission and domination. Because of the extreme closeness, the woman may also experience heightened physical sensations of deep penetration and clitoral stimulation, and may need to take breaks from the intense closeness of lovemaking. Don't let this worry either of you; some of the best sex sessions are those where couples talk, laugh, and fool around, without feeling they have to "get on with it."

• LEISURELY SEX
The best sex feels timeless and, in order to make it so, it is worth remembering a couple of points. Firstly, try to arrange to have sex at a time of day when you are not tired. If you have more energy you can pay more attention to foreplay and erotic massage, before enjoying leisurely sex. Secondly, make sure your lovemaking session is open-ended, so you can become absorbed in what you are doing and don't feel rushed. Prolong the pleasure of intimacy by continuing to caress, stroke, and massage each other in addition to, and during, sex. A good lover takes time to continue to stroke his or her partner even during the thrust of intercourse. And giving yourselves time for intimacy nurtures your physical and emotional relationship.

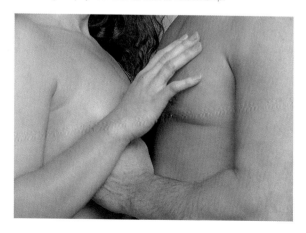

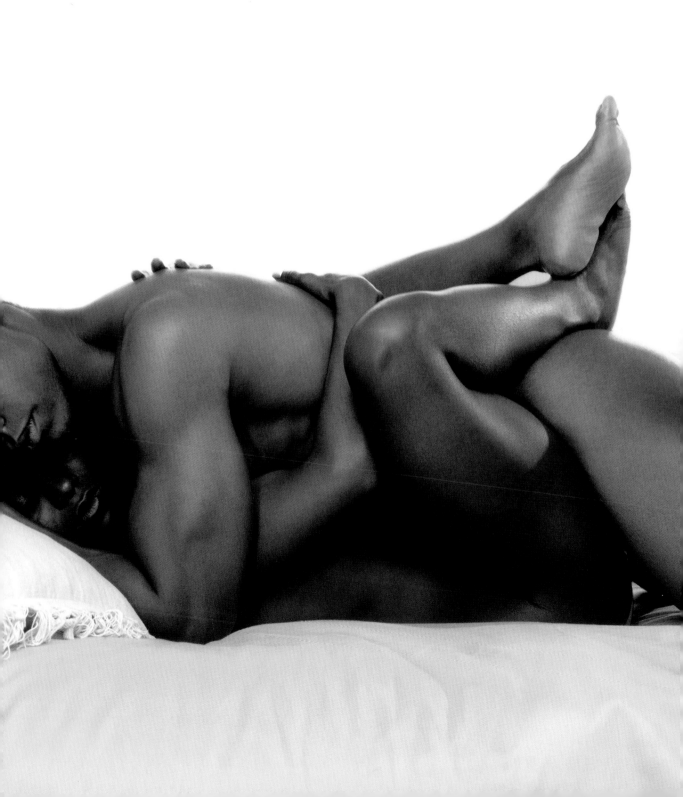

intimate wraparound

Man-on-top sexual positions have long been favored by men and women. They are comfortable, conserve energy, and are among the positions in which a woman is most likely to climax.

The woman lies on her back and raises her knees. Her partner lies on top of her, and leans forward onto his elbows and knees to support his weight. To increase the sense of intimacy, the woman crosses her ankles behind his back. In this position, she can lift and lower her hips in rhythm with his thrusts.

The man uses his toes to push against the bed as he thrusts, using his buttocks to control the power and rhythm of penetration. This vigorous action maximizes pleasure for both partners, and by lifting and spreading her thighs wide open the woman exposes her clitoris to his powerful, rhythmic stimulation.

In this position, the man can use his greater strength to control his thrusting, and so vary the pace and tempo of stimulation. This means that lovemaking can be long and drawn out, or rapid and explosive.

The woman hangs onto her man by wrapping her arms round him and keeps her ankles tightly crossed above his buttocks. This allows her to stay close to him, and move in rhythm with him to increase stimulation on her clitoris as he penetrates deeper. This is an intensely romantic position, and the perfect way to reconnect emotionally to your lover, so take the opportunity to kiss, caress, and talk tenderly to each other while making love. The physical intimacy of this erotic embrace, and the sight of the emotions on each other's faces, will greatly increase your pleasure, and may lead to more intense orgasms.

• CLITORAL STROKING

Before penetration, let your hand explore your woman's labia, stroking over her bumps and folds. This is an exciting preliminary, a promise of things to come. Next, move on to stimulating her more fully. Don't expect her genitals to be automatically moist. If they aren't, coat your fingers with saliva or lubricant. When she gets wet, step up the action by gently twirling a lubricated finger lightly on the head of the clitoris. Rub your finger on one side of her clitoris then on the other several times. Rub backward and forward immediately beneath the clitoris, then rub slowly up from underneath the clitoris right over the head. Rub across the head from one side to the other. You may also want to try out some of the genital massage techniques on pages 70–71.

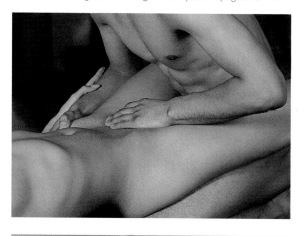

• ANGLES OF PENETRATION

The woman's sexual response during face-to-face intercourse immediately increases if her man uses his penis to put pressure on the "2 o'clock" and "10 o'clock" hot spots inside her vagina. Use a pillow under her bottom to raise her hips a little higher, and so make it easier to stimulate these pleasurable pressure points.

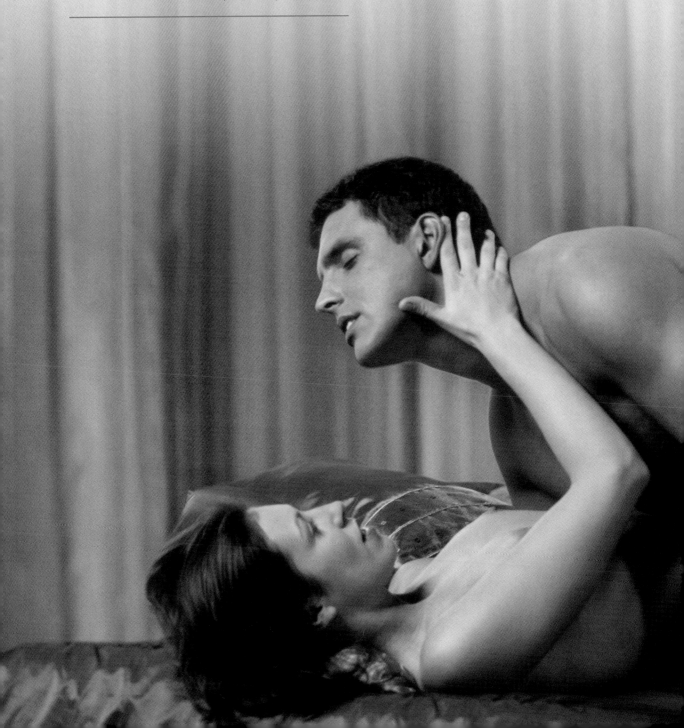

pressing together

Slide in and out of each other's embrace for languid lovemaking

Human touch has vital life-affirming and life-enhancing properties. Thus it makes sense to believe that lovers relate better if they adore holding each other tight.

The "legs entwined" position (see page 14) leads naturally into this pressing position, with the thrilling result that every part of the body feels alive. As the excitement builds between the couple, the man lowers himself closer to his partner, and is able to thrust deeper into her.

The woman grips her partner with her thighs so that her vagina and pelvic muscles tighten around his penis. The man can support himself on both knees and one arm, freeing up his other arm to stimulate her if she wants.

Value the body contact this position offers, for in terms of arousal you both will come alive. As you react to each other's intimate touch, your skin may tingle as the tension in your muscles mounts until climax.

maximum closeness

Arouse all your lover's senses with a full-body embrace

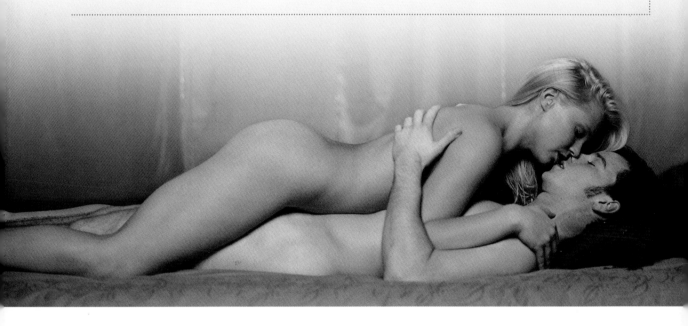

There is a lot to be said for resting on top of your man, and enjoying the long, naked closeness of each other's bodies. Kissing and whispering to each other during sex can create sensual intimacy and arousal.

This collapsed woman-on-top position is perfect for taking a rest from a more vigorous upright position. Being in control of lovemaking may greatly increase her excitement, and allow her to get very creative with movement that pleasures you both.

Here, the man lies back with his partner on top of him. She inserts his penis into her vagina, presses her breasts to his chest, and moves her hips. She can

steady herself by holding onto him. To keep his erection going, she rocks gently from side to side, until she is ready to swivel back upright again. Her swiveling hips produce a kind of churning, side-by-side movement, like a vigorous body massage, that feels very different from the usual thrust of intercourse.

• SEXY STROKES FOR HER
Stroking your woman's bottom softly can feel deeply sensual and erotic. Gently pulling her buttocks apart with both hands stretches the perineum—full of sensitive nerve endings—and gives her deep sensations of pleasure. So, too, can spanking her lightly with the flat of your hand. Gentle spanking that stings slightly arouses the blood and makes the body tingle. It can also be exciting when it comes as a surprise, as long as it is done gently.

lover's grip

Vary the angle of penetration for deeply pleasurable sensations

• SIGNS OF AROUSAL

In most men and women, the signs of sexual arousal are easy to spot: the nipples harden, muscles tense, and the feet arch and curl. When highly aroused, women usually experience a sex flush (a reddening of the skin) that starts on the throat and spreads to the breasts as her excitement heightens. In men, the sex flush begins on the belly, then spreads upward to cover the chest, neck, and face.

In this intensely intimate position, the woman raises her legs so her man can penetrate. Her openess allows him to thrust deeply, putting pressure on her clitoris and deep inside her vagina.

The man kneels, places his lover's legs over his shoulders, and raises her hips slightly to penetrate. Most men find the sexual friction and deep penetration of this position particularly exciting. During lovemaking he can use his hands to caress and stroke her legs, breasts, and to stimulate her clitoris as he thrusts.

In response, she may find that she climaxes from the powerful sensations created by his penis pressing against the walls of her vagina at different angles.

This is an exciting and innovative position for both partners but, as with any deep penetration, begin fondling and stroking well before intercourse, as she will only enjoy this position if she is properly aroused.

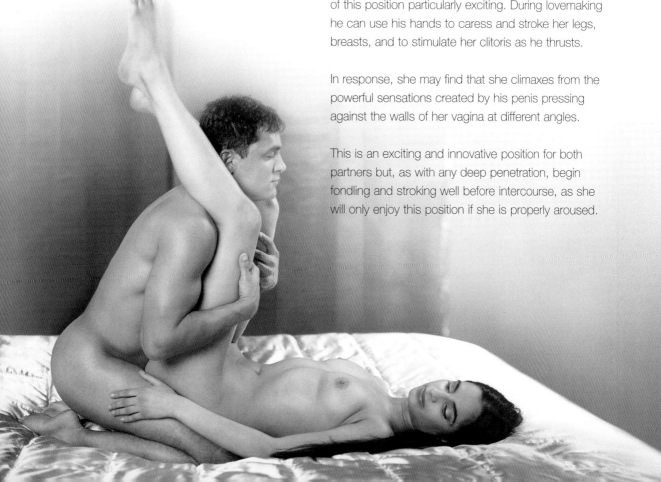

• THE EROTIC DANCE

Taoist sex educationalists specialize in teaching the art of delaying orgasm. A key premise of their teaching is that couples don't have to get stuck in the same position once sex has begun. There is nothing to stop you from moving from one position to many others in a beautiful, fluid, erotic dance.

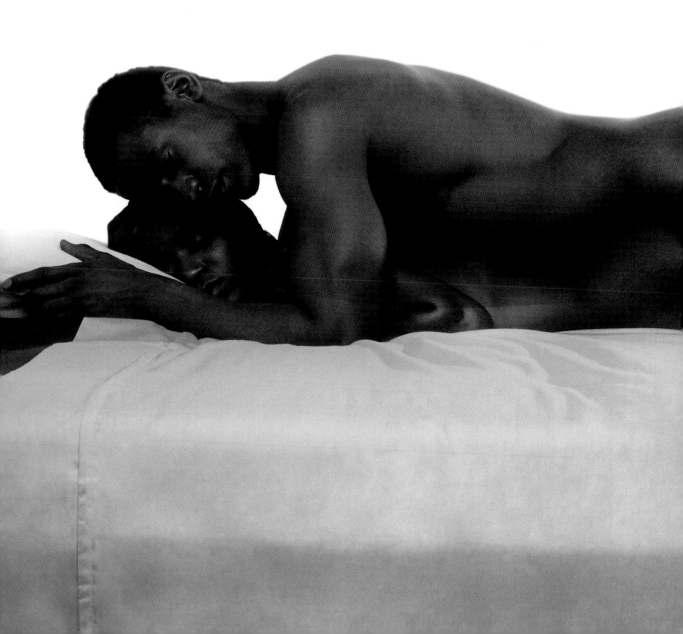

face down

Indulge in leisurely, rhythmic, and sensuous sex

This is an especially affectionate love position because the man's entire body is spread out along his partner's, with his head next to hers. Enjoy feeling the length of each other's naked bodies, kissing and whispering sexy sweet-nothings while you make love.

In this position the male pelvis rests on her buttocks, and pivots from that angle. However, because of the weight lying on top of her, the woman can't move her hips freely, and so is unlikely to gain very much clitoral pleasure from this coupling. Nor is it easy for the man to stimulate her genitals from underneath with his hands, since the weight of both bodies tends to prevent him from moving his hands easily.

Men: use this position for those times when your woman feels like taking a more passive role, or as a follow-up position when she has climaxed already, but wants to continue enjoying the intimacy of lovemaking.

Women: even if you are taking a more submissive role, make sure that you give your partner some kind of indication that he or she is having an impact: moan, sigh, kiss, and say "I love you," as the mood takes you.

kissing, licking, biting

Using your mouth to tantalize and excite your lover is one of the most intimate forms of contact human beings can experience. With a kiss, the senses of touch, taste, and smell are evoked, and this combination produces strong feelings of emotion in both giver and receiver. Licking your partner's body creates a sensual experience for you both. And when you give your lover a gentle bite on the shoulder or the neck, you express your excitement at their touch in a manner guaranteed to stoke their passion.

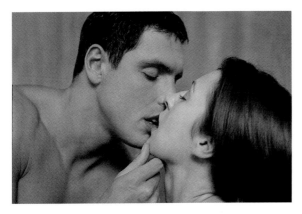

Start your kissing slowly, using your lips and hands simultaneously to express tenderness, and create a sensual build up to deeper, more passionate kisses.

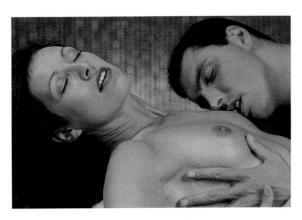

Gentle, tender kisses on your partner's breasts and nipples can be very sensual and loving. During sex, kissing her breasts may heighten her erotic experience.

Kissing the lips

A kiss can range from a quick brush of the lips to deep penetration with the tongue. The most intense kisses occur when tongues penetrate lips during lovemaking in a matching rhythm.

Experiment with different kisses at different moments to convey your feelings, from affection and adoration to lust and desire. Opt for slow kissing during foreplay, and let your kissing build as your passion grows. More urgent kisses will heighten your partner's anticipation.

Kissing the body

Gentle kisses around your partner's throat and neck often lead on naturally from lip kissing. Brush your partner's skin with soft kisses, and lavish attention on their most sensitive areas, such as the chest or breasts.

Use little staccato kisses, in which you apply your lips to the skin then quickly pull away, to show playfulness, and affection. You might scatter these across your partner's buttocks or thighs. Or give your lover a smooching progression of kisses along their spine.

You can also use your lips to apply gentle pressure by holding your mouth on their body for a moment. Make it feel as if you are almost reluctant to withdraw your lips, as you drink in the taste and smell of their skin.

Licking and biting

Being licked by your lover can feel intensely erotic, especially close to the genitals. Some areas of the body are more sensitive to the softness and wetness of the tongue than others. While you are treating your partner to an all-over licking session, don't forget to use your lips and hands from time to time, as well as your tongue, to increase the range of sensations.

Pay special attention to the breasts and nipples, the insides of the thighs, and the backs of the knees to heighten the sense of anticipation. The greater the self-control you practice as you delay sex with this artful foreplay, the richer the rewards when you move on to penetration.

Using your teeth to gently bite your lover during lovemaking heightens the intensity of the moment, while nibbling your partner's body feels erotic to both giver and receiver. The inside of the thigh is particularly sensitive, so try concentrating your teeth here. Breasts and nipples are also sensitive to being gently bitten.

Lovers might also enjoy giving and receiving love bites. This is when the skin is gently sucked using the lips and teeth to leave a mark.

....

Use your tongue, lips, and breath to tantalize and arouse your lover's erogenous zones. Use soft, firm tongue strokes to work your way down his body.

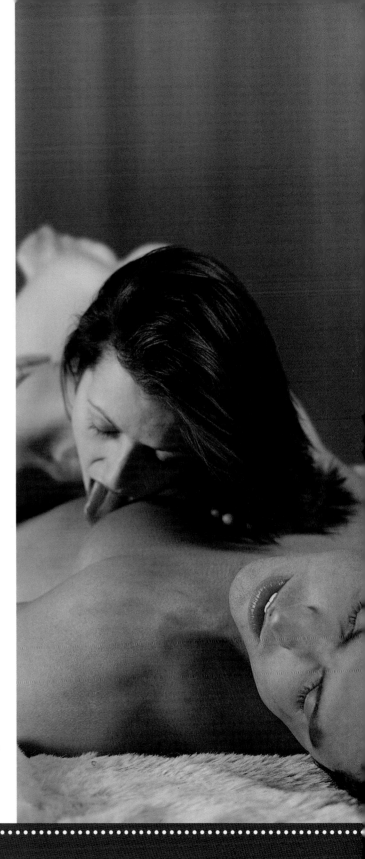

arms outstretched

Maximize vaginal stimulation in this woman-on-top position

There are many advantages to woman-on-top positions. They allow her to be a more active participant and retain control over sex, enabling her to set the tempo, movement, and depth of penetration.

In this face-to-face position the movements of the woman's outstretched arms evoke a fluttering butterfly. Here, the woman lies on top of her lover and, when she has lowered herself onto his penis, both partners stretch out their arms to either side, and hold hands.

Women: push your toes against your man's feet to move up and down. This movement increases sexual friction, and provides your man with thrilling sensations as his penis moves inside your vagina. To create intense stimulation on his frenulum, wiggle your hips and squeeze your vaginal muscles tight.

This is an enduringly intimate position, allowing couples to kiss and talk during sex. Since his movement is limited, it is a relaxing pose for when he's feeling tired, or when she wants to show her tenderness.

• INTRODUCE NOVELTY
Couples who complain that sex is boring are often asked by their therapists to try doing something fractionally different the next time they make love, such as lying on the side of the bed that their partner normally occupies. The aim of this exercise is to bring novelty into the equation, however small.

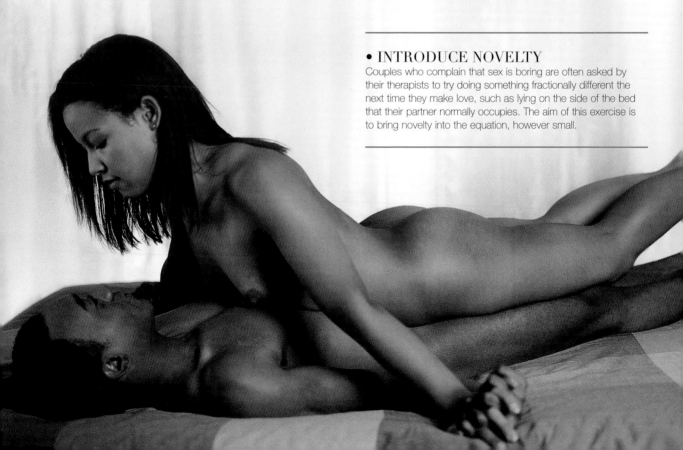

erotic flick

Excite each other with this tantalizingly slow, sensual technique

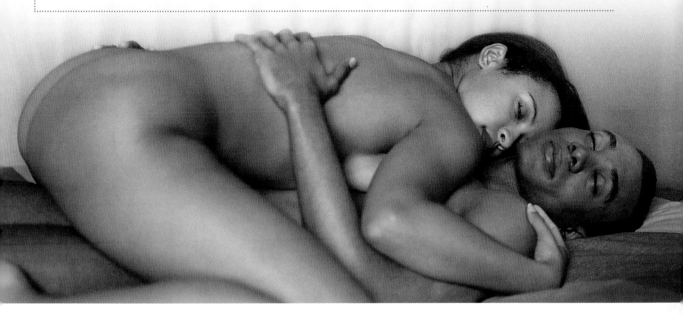

The erotic flick is so named because the woman's movements of her hips during lovemaking mimic the flick of a fish's tail as it darts through the water.

In this passive and restful position, the couple enjoy an intimate embrace as her breasts press against his chest. The woman moves her hips sensuously to pleasure him, while retaining control of lovemaking.

The man lies on his back with his legs extended as she lies on top of him. She moves forward a little, and takes in the tip of her man's penis with her labia. She uses her hands to gently position his penis then slowly wiggles it inside her. Once she has enclosed him, the

couple can nestle against each other and kiss as she moves her hips to the right and left, and up and down, in a repeated sequence.

Women: change the tempo of your movement to draw out your lover's arousal. The more excitement you build up, the greater his climax when it finally arrives.

• PHEROMONES

Men and women secrete pheromones: natural scent chemicals that serve to attract a sexual mate. Pheromones travel through the air and are drawn into our systems via our sense of smell. To make the most out of your natural chemicals, don't mask your scent with heavy perfume or soap.

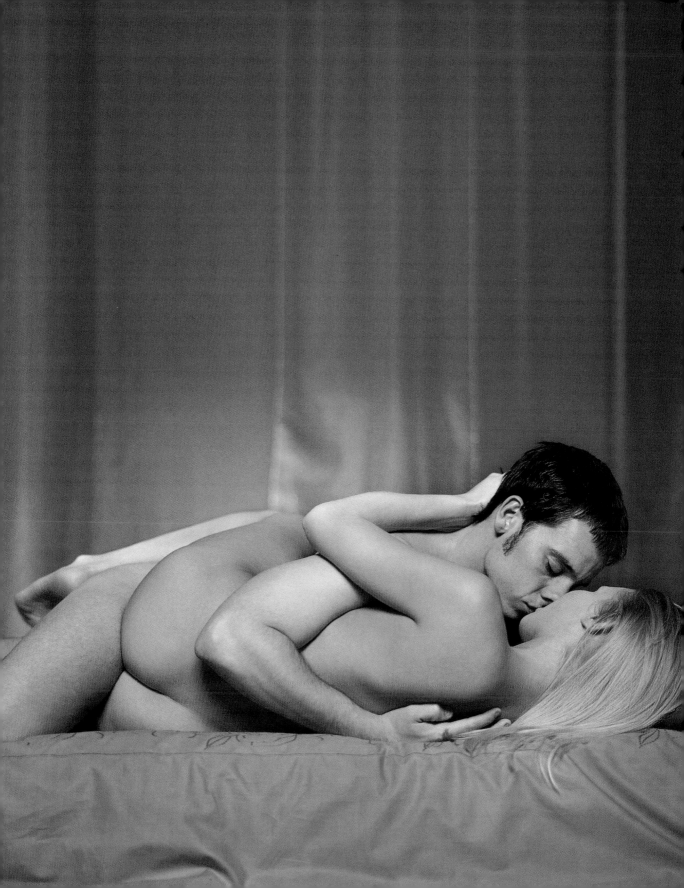

legs intertwined

Create an intimate mood that inspires feelings of tenderness

Adoring couples naturally find themselves kissing, snuggling up, and murmuring loving words, and doing this face-to-face is always more intimate and meaningful than back-to-back.

As with most side-by-side positions, this position is sensual and intimate. One of the sexiest sensations in bed is of stretching out and casually winding your legs around those of your partner. The legs, particularly the inner thighs, are full of sensitive nerve endings. Stroking each other can bring on delicate prickles of exquisite sensuality so use your hands to caress each other before penetration.

Here, both lovers lie with their legs outstretched. The woman rests her uppermost leg on top of her man's leg, bending it a little to allow him to enter her deeply. He pulls her toward him by grasping her hip, and rolling her on to her side. By pulling her, and then letting go a little, he rocks her on and off his penis.

In this way, the man can thrust vigorously to gain deep stimulation and satisfaction. As his right arm is free, he can also slide his hand up and down her neck, back, and buttocks with sensitive caresses. Her right arm can curve underneath his neck and around his shoulders in a gesture of intimacy, leaving her left arm free to roam across his body. This is an easy method of enjoying energetic sex if she is not feeling strong.

It also avoids putting weight on her abdomen, making it suitable during pregnancy. To increase her arousal, she might move in rhythm with his thrusting, and caress his genitals and buttocks to increase his feelings of excitement. This position is also recommended as a good way of slowing down orgasm.

• ALL-OVER MANUAL MASSAGE

Men are sensual creatures who enjoy receiving physical attention. Devote yourself to arousing him before sex with an all-over-body massage. Aim for maximum, whole body contact with your lover by lying down next to him naked, and using lazy, laid-back strokes. Snuggle up against him, and stroke his abdomen with one hand, and his penis with the other. Slide one hand across his chest paying special attention to his nipples while making sliding strokes on his penis. Combine penis stroking and muscle kneading along his shoulders and neck for pure sensual pleasure. The coronal ridge (the area below and around the head) is usually the most sensitive part of the penis, so whatever your strokes, make sure you stimulate this area.

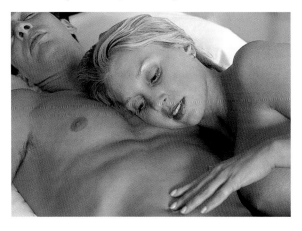

---

close curl up

Sex creates some very primitive feelings in couples, particularly the desire to get as close as possible to your lover. This position is comforting because it satisfies the need for extreme closeness.

This position is best used in combination with "puppy-love" (see page 35) to give you both a respite from intense stimulation. Here, the woman kneels with her head and arms resting on the bed while the man leans over her, and penetrates her from behind.

Men will enjoy the proximity of this position. He can drink in the scent of her skin as he kisses and nuzzles her neck. Using a combination of grinding and thrusting strokes can lead to an intense orgasm.

Although it is seductive and comfortable for her, this may not be the sexiest position. To increase the sexual friction and sensations for both of you, she can press her thighs together and clench and unclench her vaginal muscles in rhythm with his thrusts. She can also reach down and stimulate her clitoris.

• RESTING

There is no rule that specifies once you have begun thrusting you must continue all the way to climax. Try resting during intercourse, pausing to enjoy the feeling of being inside your lover, without losing your erection. This is a good way to train yourself to last longer during lovemaking.

intense intimacy

Slide into this intimate and erotic rear-facing position

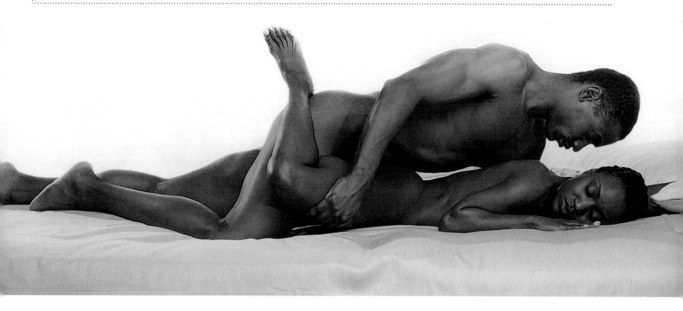

Many of the rear-facing positions are not too good for stimulating the woman's clitoris, but here the man lifts her leg from the knee to open and stretch her vagina slightly, to increase her clitoral arousal.

In this position, the woman relaxes on her front and her man lies on top of her, supporting himself on one arm and one knee. He lifts her leg gently, and then penetrates deeply from behind her.

He can choose to press his chest against her back or arch his back inward as he thrusts deeply. The animalistic power this affords him will add to his excitement and pleasure. She will enjoy the intense

intimacy given by the weight of her partner holding her down, as well as the vigorous action and deep penetration that his thrusts offers.

Her raised leg means she can also stimulate herself further by slipping her fingers between her legs to massage her clitoris, or by using a vibrator.

• SWEET MURMURS

Tender talk is a great aphrodisiac. As you make love, tell your partner how attractive you find him or her, and how much their scent or taste turns you on. Giving positive feedback to your lover raises their self-esteem, and helps them become more aware of your sexual needs and what turns you on. So, if you're enjoying his or her attentions, show your appreciation verbally.

cushioned comfort

Nuzzle her shoulders, and enjoy sensationally deep penetration

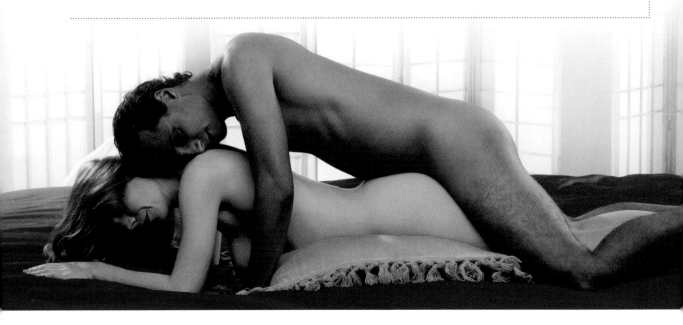

Sex from the rear is exciting because it feels good and contains a taste of the forbidden, and so ties neatly into erotic games of submission and domination.

Both sexes usually enjoy rear-entry positions—many women adore it because it makes them feel helpless, while men tend to love it because it puts them in charge. But in this variation, the women is able to take a more active role, and so gain more pleasure.

Here, the man raises himself up on his arms, enabling his woman to freely gyrate against his penis, putting her clitoris in contact with it. To avoid bruising her ribs,

and improve the angle of penetration, he can slip a cushion under her chest. For him, the sensation of thrusting below her buttocks will be a turn-on.

Men: to give your woman's clitoris more stimulation, use a grinding rather than thrusting technique, which involves vigorously pushing and circling your penis inside her vagina without actually moving in and out.

• STIMULATE YOURSELF
Many women don't get enough clitoral stimulation from rear-entry sex. In this position, it is possible to reach down and stimulate yourself with your hands to help bring you to orgasm, or use a clitoral vibrator, worn on the man's penis (see pages 164–165).

puppy love

Caress each other to orgasm in this exciting and classic position

Puppy love is a classic rear-entry pose that makes for raunchy lovemaking, while still allowing the couple to get close enough to exchange intimate kisses.

It calls for the man to kneel as he thrusts into his partner from behind. Since both partners are kneeling, she can use her arms to steady herself against his thrusting, yet raise her body up easily for closer, more intimate contact with him.

This provocative pose gives him easy access to her clitoris, while allowing him to control the tempo of his thrusts. He can add to her excitement by reaching down between her legs and using a fingertip to gently massage her clitoris during lovemaking; it's a very effective way of exciting her, and can bring her to orgasm. He will also enjoy the sensations of being able to thrust freely while still being able to stroke her breasts and kiss her neck.

In return, the woman opens her legs wide, and arches her back to allow him to penetrate her deeply. Rearing up like this, she can choose to stimulate herself or use a vibrator (see pages 164–165). Pushing her pelvis toward him will increase penetration, while moving away from him can make his thrusts shallower.

Women: to delay his orgasm, try reaching back between his legs and gently tugging on his testicles. This can slow him down at the crucial moment.

• STROKING YOURSELF

This is a perfect position for the woman to stroke herself. Revel in the sensations you arouse beneath your fingers—start by caressing your breasts and nipples, then move on to fondling your pubic area, letting your hands stray around the inner thighs, then gently explore the outer labia. Try out different strokes of varying pressure, to find out what feels best.

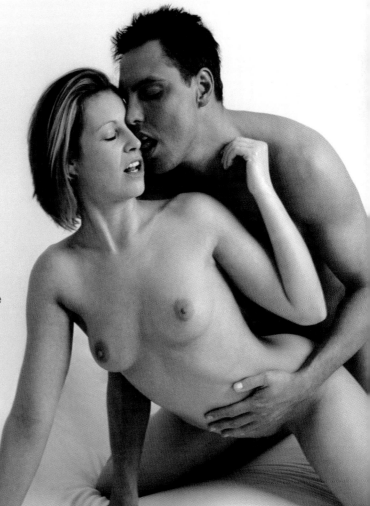

• LOCATING HER G-SPOT
To locate your woman's G-spot, insert your forefinger into her vagina, and rest your fingertip on the front wall about two-thirds of the way along her vagina toward the cervix. Her G-spot feels like a muscular crossroads, a small configuration of muscles that is able to resist firm but gentle pressure from your fingertip. Continued pressure can, in some women, lead to an orgasm.

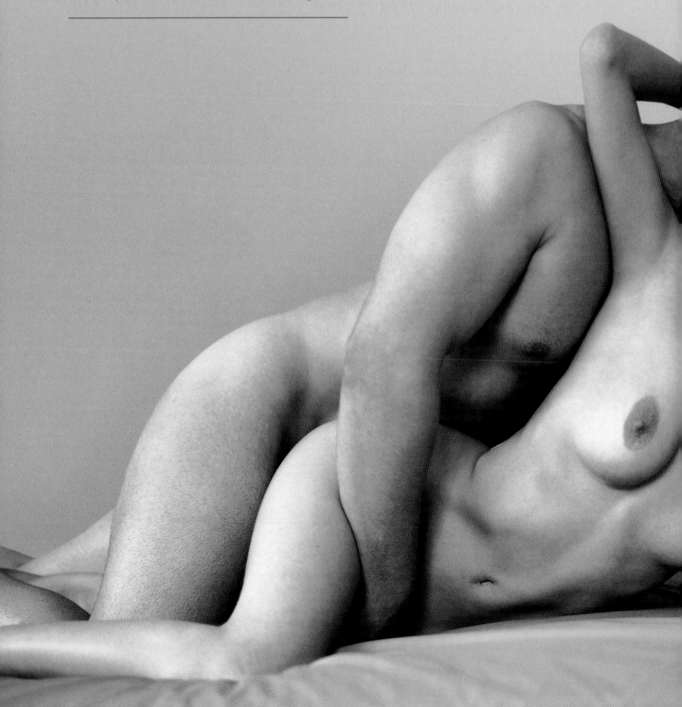

lovers' vine

Revel in the **sensations** of turning and twining around each other

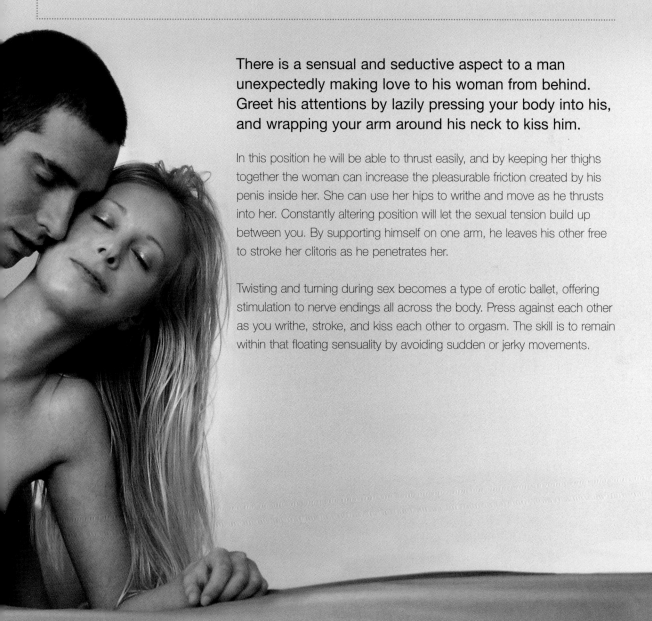

There is a sensual and seductive aspect to a man unexpectedly making love to his woman from behind. Greet his attentions by lazily pressing your body into his, and wrapping your arm around his neck to kiss him.

In this position he will be able to thrust easily, and by keeping her thighs together the woman can increase the pleasurable friction created by his penis inside her. She can use her hips to writhe and move as he thrusts into her. Constantly altering position will let the sexual tension build up between you. By supporting himself on one arm, he leaves his other free to stroke her clitoris as he penetrates her.

Twisting and turning during sex becomes a type of erotic ballet, offering stimulation to nerve endings all across the body. Press against each other as you writhe, stroke, and kiss each other to orgasm. The skill is to remain within that floating sensuality by avoiding sudden or jerky movements.

inverted embrace

Enjoy the long, naked sensation of each other's bodies

The rocking and resting that makes up the inverted embrace helps you maintain sexual interest while offering both of you breathing space from more vigorous sex.

Here, the woman lies full length along her partner's body with her knees on either side of his thighs, and uses her hands to support her weight. To keep him aroused, and his erection going, she squeezes his penis, and rocks gently from side to side.

Women in particular may find this position a sensual rest from more strenuous woman-on-top lovemaking. It gives both partners the chance to kiss, stroke, and nuzzle each other until she is ready to resume a more sexually exciting position.

● PEAKING

By stopping and starting stimulation, you can reach mini-peaks of climax without completely achieving orgasm. You can do this by changing tempo, position, or stopping to rest. Men and women can reach many smaller peaks before finally letting go.

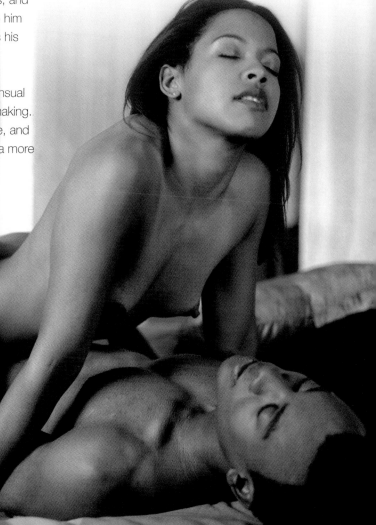

leg wrap

Get as close as you can and revel in erotic lovemaking

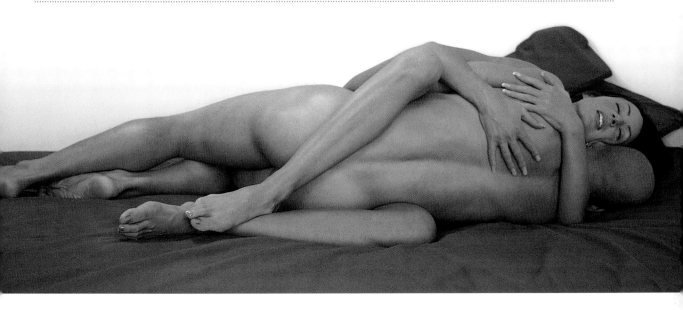

Many lovers feel aroused by the sheer sensation of wrapping their legs round each other. In this intimate position, the woman hooks both her legs directly over her lover's hips so she is wide open.

Her mobility is greatly increased during sex in this position, since wrapping her legs around her partner's buttocks allows her to thrust against his body.

He will love the feeling of tightness as she squeezes her vagina around his penis. He will also be able to penetrate deeply in this position as her open legs allow him in. Most men find being enclosed by their lover's

arms, legs, and vagina very erotic. In addition, stroking your lover's back and buttocks sends thrilling tingles of pleasure down their spine.

Women: you may find this position uncomfortable to sustain if your partner is heavier than you, so save it for when you are both ready to climax.

• THE ART OF BITING

When passion heats up, your kisses may become more urgent, and you may feel like biting your partner to show him or her your feelings. Don't be afraid to use your teeth during an embrace: it can be very sexy for the other person, and a good way of showing your appreciation. Just don't bite too hard. Aim to take your lover's skin between your teeth without breaking it.

• SEXY SIGNALS

It is probably our primitive instincts that make us become sexually excited at the sight and sensation of a mate's buttocks. Among primates, the anal region gives a focal sexual signal, and humans are almost certainly no different from their monkey cousins. It is a good reason why cuddling in the spoons position brings on a regular reaction—that of becoming quickly turned on. The great advantage of having sex while lying down is that it conserves energy, whatever your health or well-being.

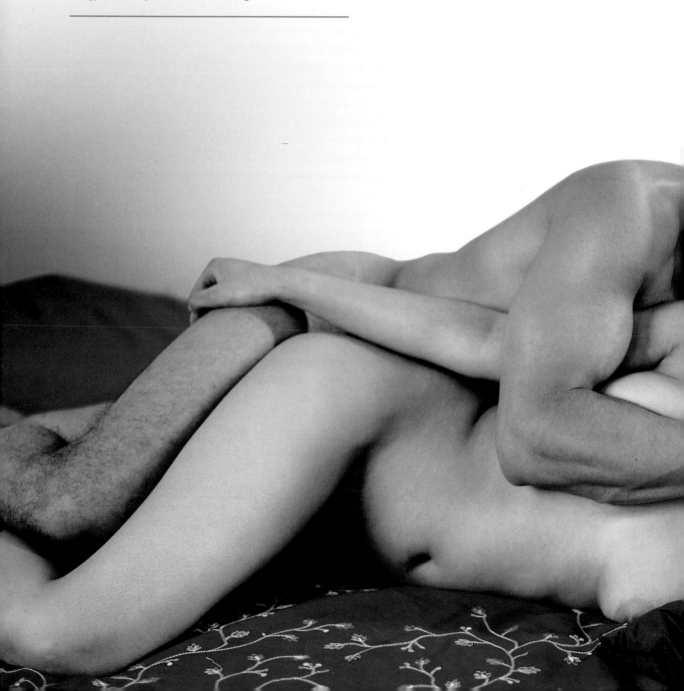

spoons

Absorb yourselves in each other's bodies with all-over contact

This position is erotic and romantic as expanses of your naked skin rub together. When the man cuddles up closely to the woman's buttocks from behind, it is often a great turn-on for both partners, and leads easily to the start of intimate lovemaking.

In the classic spoons position, the woman lies on her side while the man presses up tightly against her back and penetrates her gently from the rear, keeping his movements shallow. He can turn her chest and head toward him, so he and his partner can kiss and whisper to each other.

It is the perfect position for slow, affectionate lovemaking when the woman is heavily pregnant, or for those sexy moments first thing in the morning when you are aroused but only half-conscious. Your sleepy desire will develop gradually into an energizing sexual heat of passion and orgasm. Alternatively, use this position to rediscover intimacy with your lover by taking turns to stroke each other as you make love.

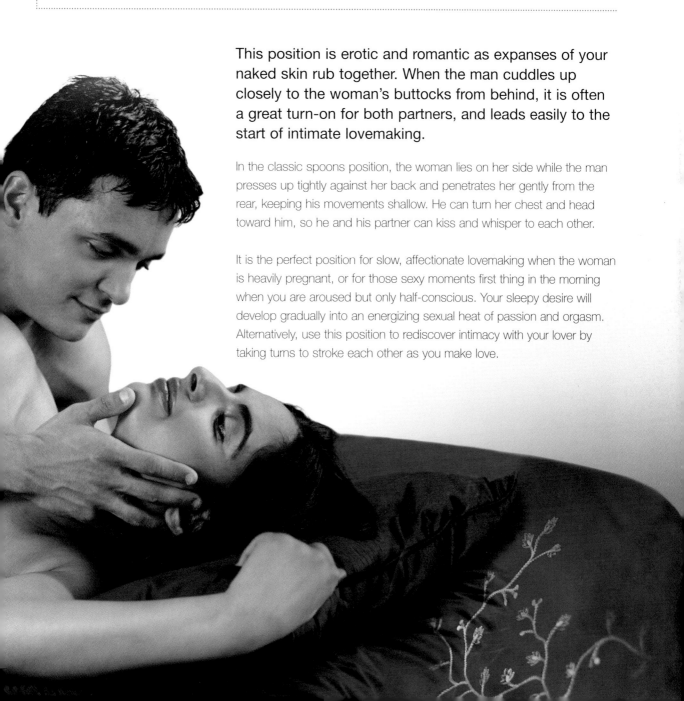

sensual massage

Touch doesn't only involve sensation—it conveys and evokes emotions and attraction, and is the foundation for love. It is such a primitive form of connection that the minute you are touched reassuringly, you feel better. When someone caresses your body, your ego is stroked too. And the person giving the caress feels good, because he or she is also experiencing the physical and emotional contact of touch. Massage is the perfect precursor to sex, and couples often find that lovemaking follows on naturally from it.

Sensual preparations

Before you start your massage, wash your hands in hot water, so that they feel warm and clean. Make sure the room is warm, and create a clear space. The floor is the best place for a massage, and you can make the area more comfortable for your partner by laying some bath towels over a rug. Now, pour a little warmed massage oil into each hand, then rub your hands together to give each palm a liberal coating. Start by using slow, continuous movements, so that you have at least one hand in contact with your partner's body at all times.

Circling

There are several different massage strokes, but the most useful one is "circling." You can give an effective and sensual all-over body massage using circling alone.

To circle, place both hands, palms down, then move them firmly in opposing circles. You can make large, wide circles, small, delicate circles, or something in between. Don't circle on bony areas. Circle with both hands on either side of the spine, massaging away from the spine – never toward it or on it. Circling can be used to

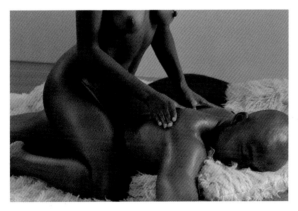

Giving a naked massage means that your partner gets the benefit of your hands, and the erotic sensations that your naked, oiled body creates against his or her body.

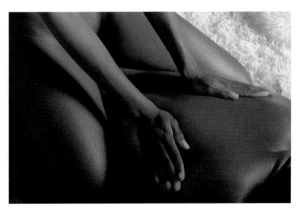

Give an all-over massage by moving your hands in large and small circles. Start at the shoulders, go down to the buttocks and back up again. Keep it slow and sensual.

link to other strokes and other parts of the body. Try using circling strokes on your partner's back, front, hands, feet, face, and head.

Varying pressure

The most intense pressure is applied in "kneading," which is a very good massage stroke for getting through to the deep muscle layers of the lower back, hips, and buttocks.

To knead, use the thumb and forefingers of both hands simultaneously to rhythmically squeeze and release rolls of skin, almost as if kneading dough. Combine kneading with "thumbing" in which you make short, rapid, strokes either in circles or by pushing up against the skin for a few inches.

When your partner feels truly worked over and receptive to something a little sexier, use strokes with lighter pressure, such as "feathering". This is a playful and erotic stroke, best used after the main part of the massage.

To feather, lightly waft the fingertips of both hands in circles across your partner's body or in downward cascades of gentle strokes.

A fingertip (or even a fingernail) massage, which involves feather-light touches brushing over the surface of the skin, can be extremely exciting and erotic. But it's a good idea to do this after using the other layers of pressure first. Be careful, however, to keep your touch slow and sensual to avoid tickling your partner.

....

Vary the intensity by applying different pressures with your strokes. Begin with a firm pressure, then move into a lighter touch, and finally apply strokes with fingertips only.

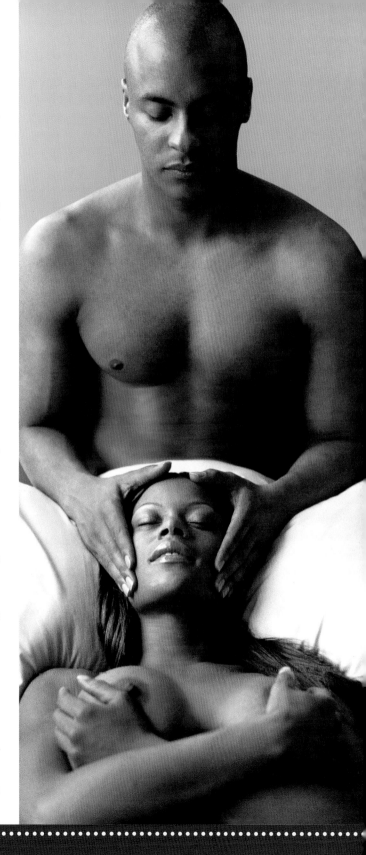

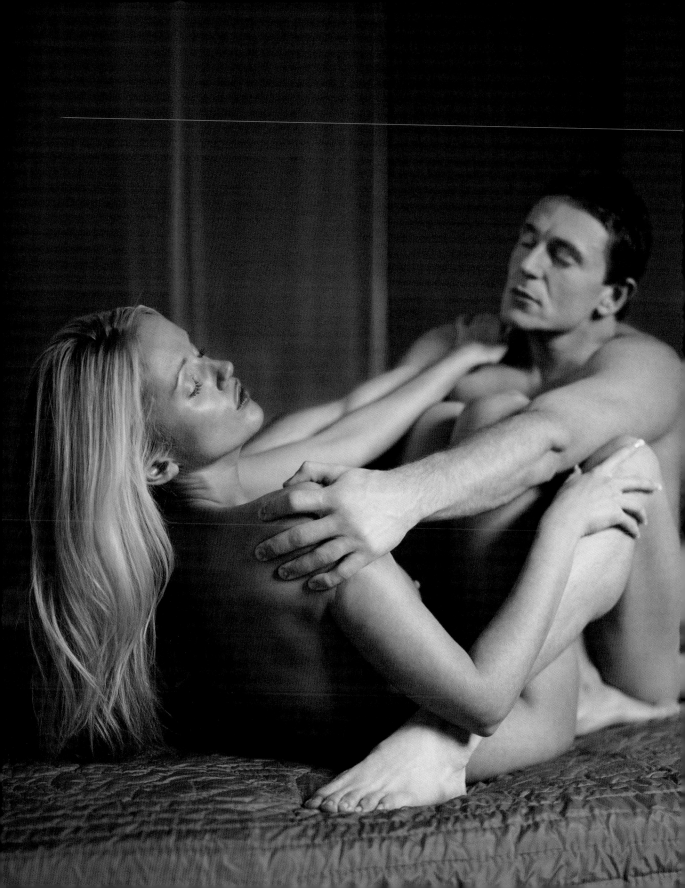

erotic squeeze

Get carried away in the moment and try something new

Use this position when you want to make love in front of the fire, or simply to spice up your usual sexual routine. The unusual rocking motion feels friendly, and inspires trust between lovers.

Here, the man sits with his knees apart, and the woman sits between his legs. The man holds onto her shoulders and pulls her forward onto his penis. He needs to push her knees back gently so that her heels are close enough to her buttocks to allow him room for entry. She wraps her arms around his knees and shoulders, and leans back as she squeezes her vaginal muscles to grip his penis. Since her feet are tucked underneath his buttocks, she can lean back with quite a degree of comfort and push against him.

To enjoy stimulation and climax in this position, the couple needs to build up friction between them, because stimulation arises from their close, intense contact. Instead of thrusting, the man grinds against her, pushing and circling his penis inside her vagina without actually moving in and out. At the moment of orgasm, the man can grasp his lover's upper arms and draw her toward him.

Women may enjoy the physical security and intimacy of this position. It may even reveal deeper feelings of vulnerability and trust. Men will enjoy the pressure that her vagina places on his penis, while the rocking motion stimulates him and maintains his excitement.

Most couples will enjoy the novelty of this position, and it can enable both partners to build intimacy and sensation. Even though neither partner has much freedom to move in this position, the small movements cause sexual tension to mount between them, making it an excellent precursor to a more active position.

• LOVING INGREDIENTS

Old-fashioned concepts of trust and respect are vital ingredients for creating a sense of spiritual peace between long-term lovers. Many men and women possess a fragile self-confidence that can be easily knocked, and they are especially vulnerable during lovemaking. Make each other feel trusted and respected by following these simple rules. Don't criticize your partner to his or her face or behind their back. Don't ignore your partner's requests or lie to them. Do get more physical with each other and show affection. Go in for hugging, and do a lot of it. Tell him or her "I love you," at least once a day. During the day, focus on your partner at least 50 percent of the time. Be supportive of each other's pursuits in work, health, and play.

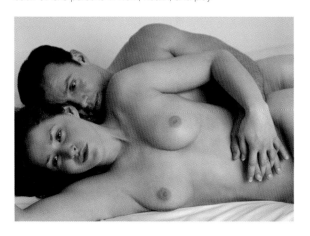

easy love

Kiss and caress each other in loving intimacy

Side-by-side lovemaking limits both lovers' freedom of movement, enabling them to focus on stroking and kissing each other while building up stimulation.

In this position, the couple lie side by side and the woman raises her leg slightly to allow her partner to enter her. He raises his leg and rests it on her thigh. Positions in which the woman has her legs closed automatically constrict the muscles and hold her labia bunched firmly against his penis.

She can squeeze her vaginal muscles to put pressure on his penis, intensifying her own pleasure and his arousal. As friction builds up between them, both partners can enjoy exquisite sensations.

If he needs especially strong friction on his penis, he may achieve greater sensation by pulling himself up slightly toward her head so that the tip of his penis almost leaves her vagina every time he pulls out of her. This will also ensure that his penis brushes against her clitoris with each stroke.

• MORE FRICTION

Side-by-side positions are excellent for men who need more friction during intercourse. The penis thrusts are felt along the insides of the labia, which are pressed against the penis by the legs, so these positions also give the woman an increased likelihood of orgasm. The combination of stroking and clitoral stimulation are very exciting for her, and side-by-side positions are often used as part of sex therapy for women who have had difficulty achieving orgasm in the past.

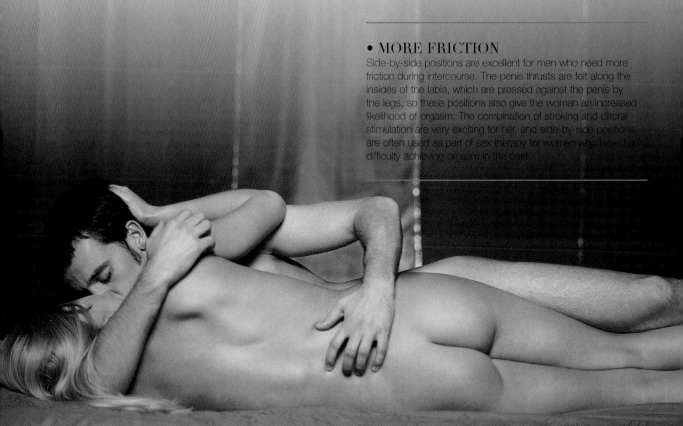

sexy snug

Get as close as possible to each other

Any face-to-face position feels erotic, especially if seated squeezed up against your lover's body. Here, both partners control the gentle rhythm of lovemaking.

The man sits on the floor, or the bed, with his knees bent wide open while his partner sits with her legs over his thighs and her feet on the floor. The couple pull each other close to enable him to penetrate. The experience is emotionally very sexy.

A gentle rocking motion rather than a thrusting action provides just enough stimulation to maintain arousal. The man can grasp her around the buttocks to help lift her as she moves up and down, while the woman can rhythmically squeeze and let go with her thighs. This pleasures him while stimulating her clitoris.

This position may not be orgasmic for either of you, but you will enjoy the experience of moving in tandem to create such a beautiful coupling.

• SWEET LOVE
If you both have a sweet tooth, treat your lover to a series of sweet tricks: hide a mint in your mouth as you kiss; tie some licorice twists around his penis then eat it; demonstrate fellatio on a lollipop or give oral sex with a mouthful of sherbert. Finish by arranging a candy trail leading to where you want to be kissed.

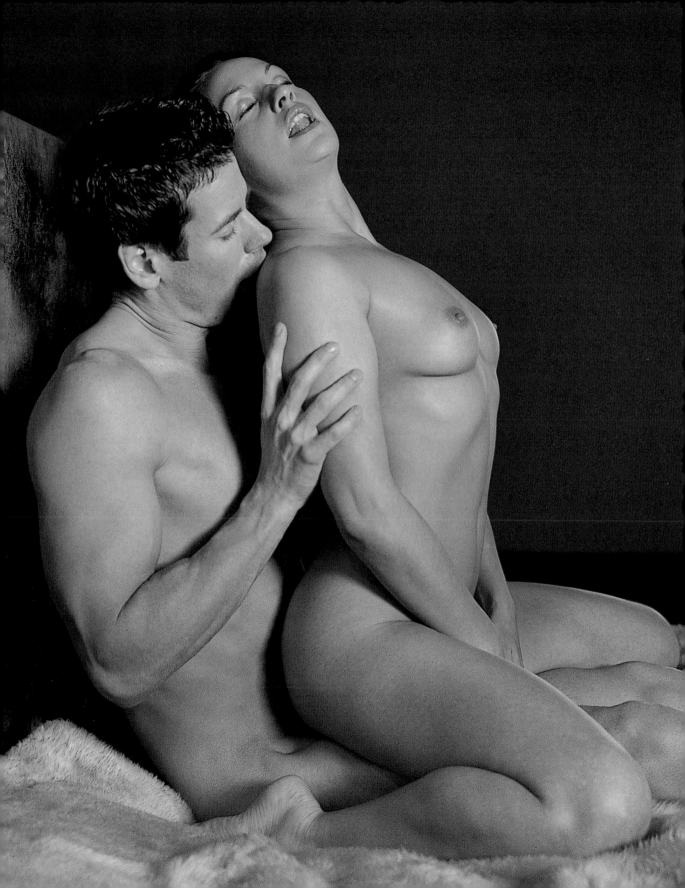

fun on top

Some of the heat is taken off the man as the woman leans into him so he can enter from the rear. The couple's heads are close enough to kiss occasionally as she rises and falls above him.

In this position, the woman sits astride the man facing away, and takes control of lovemaking. She uses her thigh muscles to rise and fall, and so sets the tempo by thrusting as she desires.

The long drawn-out sensation of her moving up and down on his penis may quickly bring him to orgasm. To slow sex down, the woman can alternate bigger thrusting movements with smaller movements in which she uses her vaginal muscles to repeatedly squeeze his penis, as if milking it.

In this position, the man has easy access to her if he wants to caress her clitoris and breasts with his hands. She can enhance his excitement by reaching between his legs to stroke and caress his inner thighs. Use your hands to caress, cup, fondle, and stroke his testicles, and to caress his perineum—the area between the anus and the testicles—which is a powerhouse of erotic sensation.

Your man might suggest this position if he is feeling unwell, incapacitated—but lustful—or just wants to play the passive role. If so, he might find it helpful to lie back against a wall propped up on a pile of cushions.

This is to provide solid support as well as comfort. It is also a good position for couples who don't always want sex to be the height of passion. Sometimes you may prefer not to have every facial flicker observed. At those times, this position feels restful and intimate while giving both partners plenty of good vibrations.

• NECK SPOTS

Many men and women will have discovered this pathway of extreme pleasure by accident when their lover has adoringly kissed or bitten them around the ear, neck, or shoulder. It's an area so sensitive that it affects arousal throughout the body, especially the genitals. To find the best place, look at the base of your partner's neck, where the back of the skull meets the top of the neck. Directly underneath the skull, on either side of the neck bones, you will find some very small muscles which may feel very tight. This area is a secret sensation source that responds to massage strokes. Massage your own neck to understand how best to massage your partner's. Go in lightly. Too much pressure on this sensitive area can hurt.

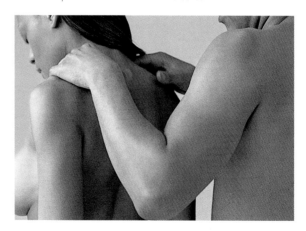

side-by-side clasping

Clasp your lover and reconnect emotionally and physically

The act of wrapping yourself lovingly around your partner stimulates every nerve ending in the body, generates feelings of tenderness and comfort, and provides a slow build-up to sex.

Here, the lovers intertwine their legs and use their hands to caress each other's bodies. In this position you both feel protected and protective. Your senses come alive as your skin is stroked, enabling you to relax and begin slow, unhurried love.

Take it easy, and explore the notion of delayed gratification in order to build up sexual tension and desire between you.

Take turns to lightly stroke and caress your partner's whole body using your fingertips only. The end result is that you both feel spoiled and loved. Ideally, you will also feel sexually charged. The loving intimacy of this side-by-side clasping embrace is reassuring and sensual, especially if either partner suffers from any anxiety associated with sex.

• PULL HIM CLOSER
Intensify your, and his, sexual excitement in this position by stopping him for an instant, and using your hands to firmly pull his buttocks toward you as he thrusts. Emotionally he will feel submerged in the sensation of being enclosed by you, while you in turn experience deep penetration.

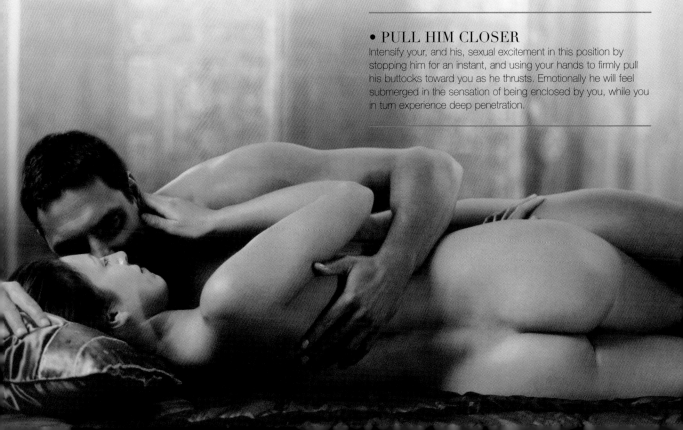

sexy embrace

Pull her toward you as she wraps her legs around you

The best sex comes spontaneously, when you and your partner pick up on each other's emotions and desires and start to create a cycle of increasing arousal.

This position brings a new angle to your lovemaking, as the woman submits to her man's desires and wraps her legs around him to get as close as possible.

She lies on her back, with her legs on either side of her man. He kneels before her and lifts her hips up to meet his penis. In this position, the woman is open to deep penetration. He supports her back with his hands as he thrusts, while she squeezes her vaginal muscles tight to hold him against her. She can reach up to fondle his neck, shoulders, and nipples.

She can draw her man even closer by crossing her ankles behind his back, emphasizing her feelings of tenderness and intimacy, and her desire to get close to him. As the man hugs the woman to him, he can slip a cushion under her back so that she can thrust against him without hurting herself, increasing pleasure for them both. An excitingly acrobatic pose!

• OIL WRESTLING

Closely tangled positions like this can be enhanced if you and your parter get oiled up. There is an extra thrill in getting totally messy and abandoning all control. Use an old shower curtain or a PVC fitted bed-sheet to oil-proof your bed or floor. Lubricate each other's bodies with any kind of oil you like: baby oil, massage oil, or olive oil, and start wriggling and writhing. Warning: don't use oils towards a latex condom, as they can weaken the latex.

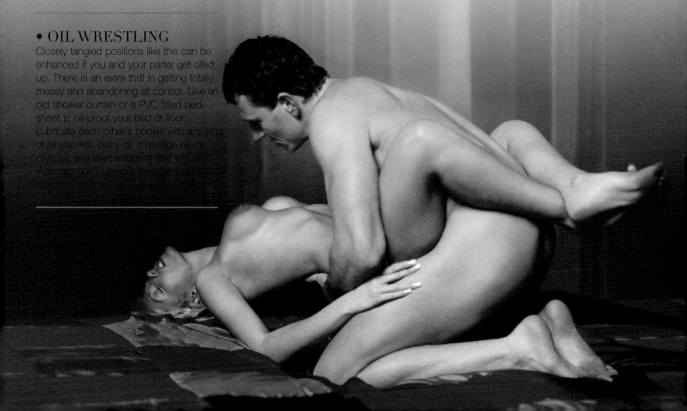

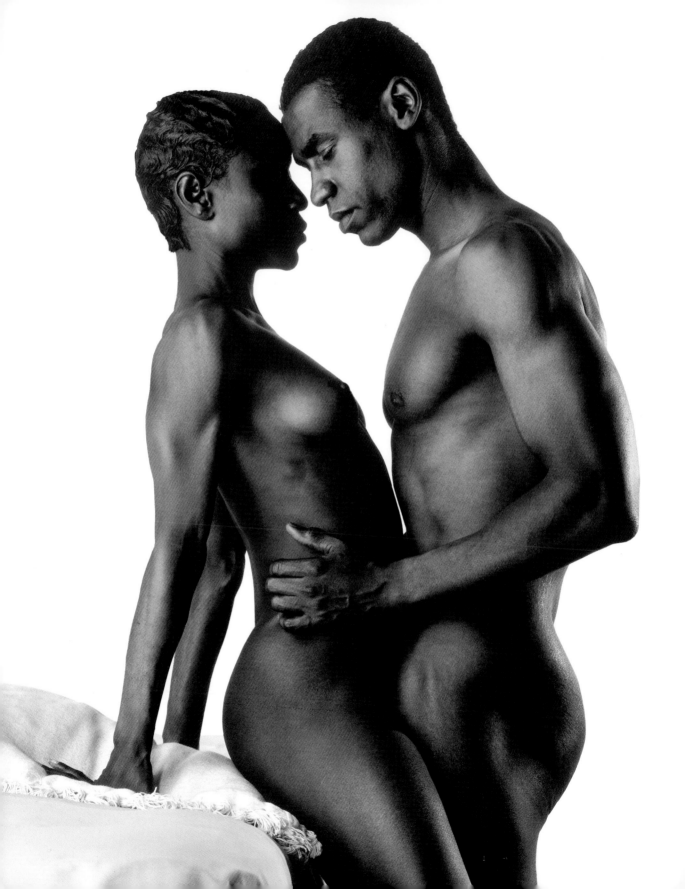

belly-to-belly

Not all face-to-face positions involve lying down. In "belly-to-belly" we find a direct, lustful, and intimate position. Just holding each other close and face-to-face when you are having sex is very sensual—especially if you are both naked.

Many men and women fantasize about having sex while standing up—possibly because they associate upright intercourse with the idea of surprise seduction. Standing positions offer the intriguing possibility of having sex anywhere or any time—the hall, on the stairs, against a wall… Making love in unconventional ways and unusual places like these opens your mind and body to new sensations, and the excitement can create fresh intimacy with your lover.

The man stands facing his woman and holds her around the waist to penetrate her. She steadies herself by leaning back with her hands on a bed or sofa. Most of the lovemaking action comes from her, but the man can help by supporting her in his arms.

As his excitement increases, he can caress and kiss her, or embrace her with his arms while letting his hands roam across her back. Since his partner may be shorter than him in height, he can bend his knees so that he can fit inside her. This is especially useful if he has a long penis. The angle of penetration will stimulate her G-spot, giving her wonderful sensations.

Every slight deviation of standing sex provides specific sensation, and special eroticism. As he thrusts, it helps if she can lift one leg upward—this opens her vagina a little more, and envelops him even further. If the woman wants to take both her legs off the ground, she might sit on a table or be supported by her man from underneath. Holding up your female partner during intercourse is a Herculean labor of love, and not one many men will manage for very long.

• ENCOURAGING INTIMACY

In a relationship feelings of intimacy can wax and wane and this is perfectly normal. However you can encourage intimacy by following these three simple guidelines. First, give and receive love by kissing and cuddling, and don't assume sex is the only sure indication that you are loved. Next, always encourage your partner, and be aware that your negative emotions can affect him or her too. Finally, suggest some practical options if your partner is having difficulty resolving a problem. This aspect of intimacy will always form part of a strong relationship.

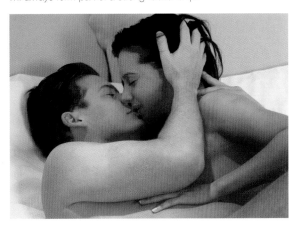

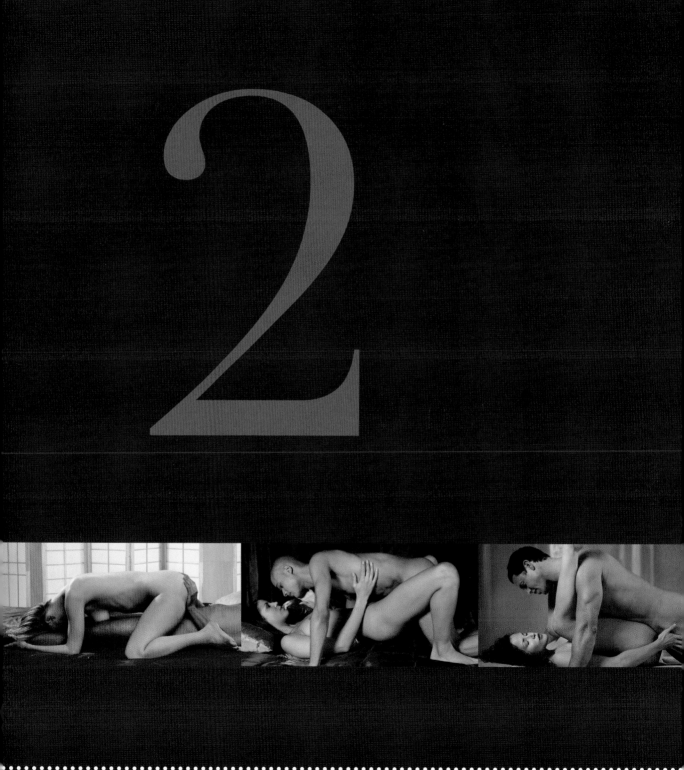

Maximum Sensation

One of the greatest mistakes lovers make is to rush through sex. Men and women do this equally because they're impatient, embarrassed, not sure what else to do, or simply can't wait any longer. But if rushing becomes routine then both lovers miss out. There are numerous ways to linger over sex, and for many you need extra time, conversation, and a a youthful ability to play.

Here is a wealth of sex techniques to help you slow down your lovemaking. Explore the secrets of delaying his orgasm in positions such as Flower in a Vase or The Grip. Pleasure each other's bodies using your mouths, lips, and tongues in Soixante-neuf. Achieve deeper penetration in The Press or Raised Feet. Find new techniques to arouse your lover in the Scissors or Sensuous Paddle.

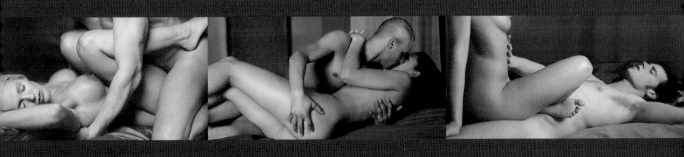

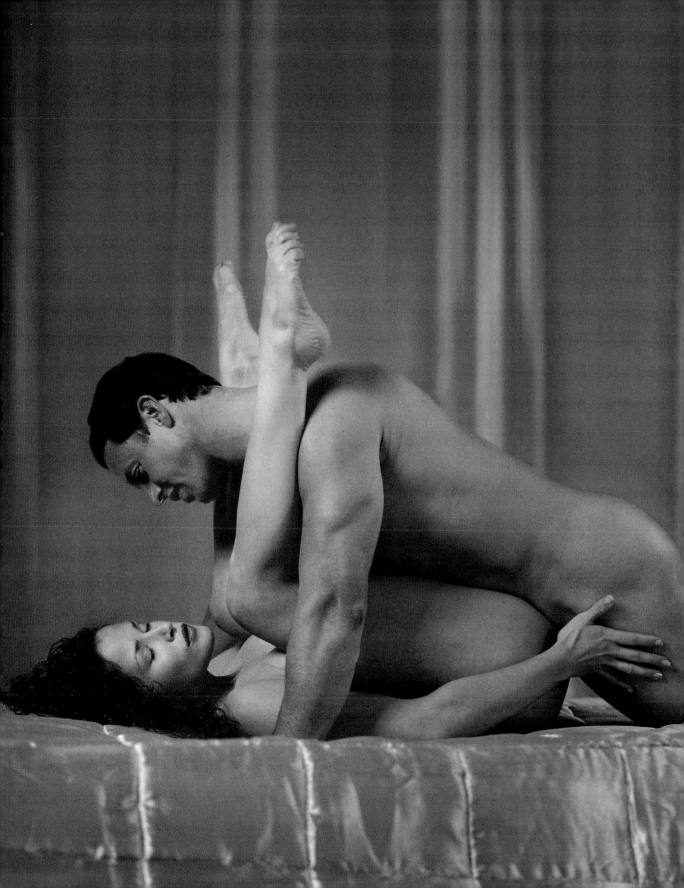

deep yawn

Lie back, and enjoy all the sensations of deep, lustful penetration

The act of raising your legs high in the air opens you up, making you feel excitingly vulnerable and erotically available. Your man also gets a buzz from being in the dominant position.

Here, the woman raises her legs and rests her calves on her man's shoulders. The man lies over his partner, supporting himself on his arms as he thrusts or rocks from a semi-upright position. The couple can watch each others' faces, and, as she holds her legs high in the air, the woman's pose adds an element of powerful eroticism to lovemaking for both partners.

The woman can increase the depth of penetration by pulling her knees as close as possible to her chest. Men should thrust very gently in this position—some women have an over-sensitive cervix, and slamming into it can shock and bruise, rather than delight your lover. Because of the extreme depth of penetration, she needs to be be fully aroused before you move into this position, or she may find it uncomfortable.

For her, the intense local sensation of the thrust and withdrawal of his penis is very sexy, even though there is no direct stimulation of her clitoris. She may also find the pressure put on her perineum and anal area is arousing. If the woman has strong core muscles, she can lift her pelvis up and the couple can use a gentle rocking motion to stimulate each other.

Be warned, this is a tiring position for the man, and it is unlikely that he will be able to sustain it for long. However, it does enable him to thrust deeply inside her, which may make up for the fatigue. If he needs to rest during lovemaking, the woman can caress his genitals and testicles until he is ready to carry on.

• INCREASE EROTICISM

Every day, tell your lover what you love about him or her, and also tell yourself what you love about you. Add to the eroticism of your lovemaking by putting mirrors alongside your bed, so you and your lover can watch yourselves making love. An extension of this idea is to record the sounds of your lovemaking, or make a movie of it. Send each other love letters, sexy texts, or leave love notes in unexpected places. Or wrap up a sexy object in beautiful paper; you might offer a bottle of massage oil, a feather boa, or an erotic picture. Describe your sexual fantasies to each other in explicit detail. Confess your desires and feelings to your partner over the phone; stimulate yourself while telling your lover that you are imagining that it's he or she who is arousing you.

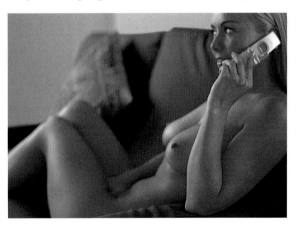

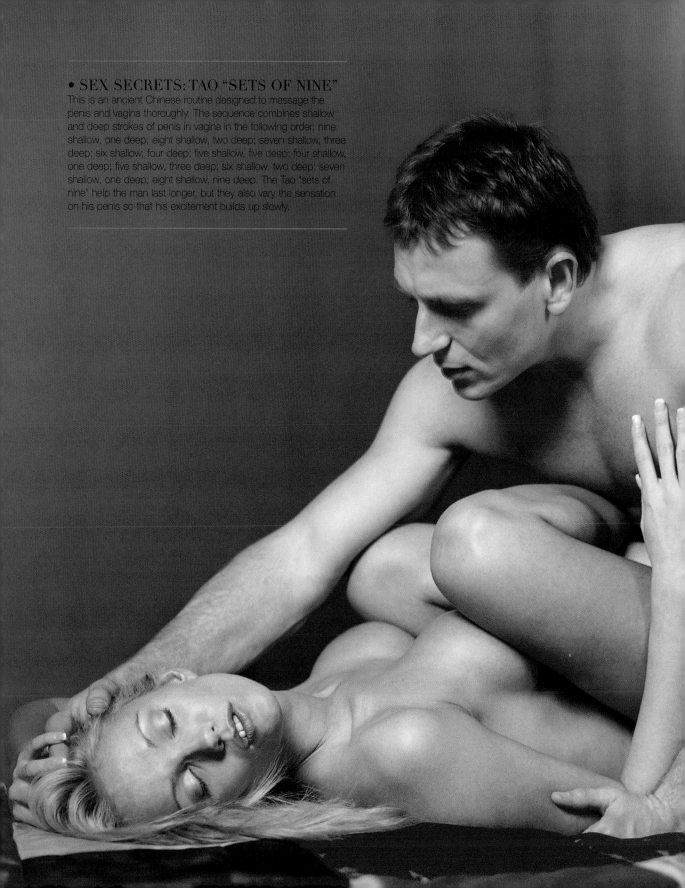

• SEX SECRETS: TAO "SETS OF NINE"

This is an ancient Chinese routine designed to massage the penis and vagina thoroughly. The sequence combines shallow and deep strokes of penis in vagina in the following order: nine shallow, one deep; eight shallow, two deep; seven shallow, three deep; six shallow, four deep; five shallow, five deep; four shallow, one deep; five shallow, three deep; six shallow, two deep; seven shallow, one deep; eight shallow, nine deep. The Tao "sets of nine" help the man last longer, but they also vary the sensation on his penis so that his excitement builds up slowly.

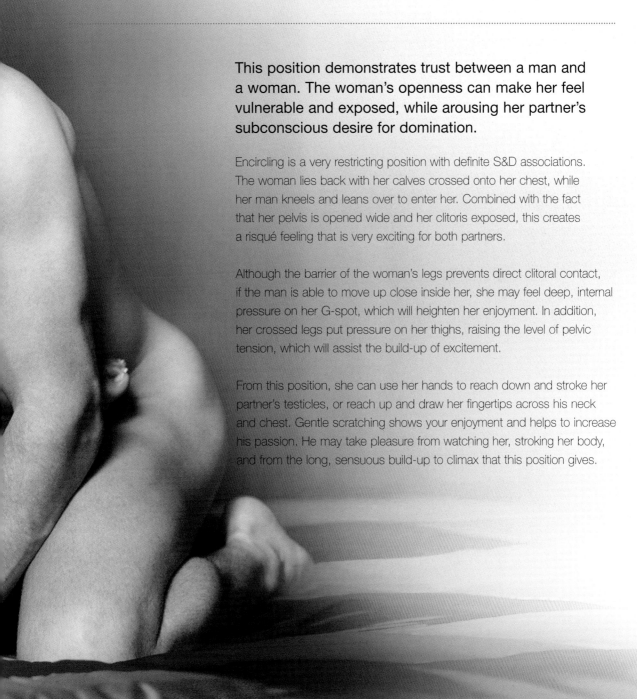

encircling

Open yourself up to the bondage-style eroticism of this pose

This position demonstrates trust between a man and a woman. The woman's openness can make her feel vulnerable and exposed, while arousing her partner's subconscious desire for domination.

Encircling is a very restricting position with definite S&D associations. The woman lies back with her calves crossed onto her chest, while her man kneels and leans over to enter her. Combined with the fact that her pelvis is opened wide and her clitoris exposed, this creates a risqué feeling that is very exciting for both partners.

Although the barrier of the woman's legs prevents direct clitoral contact, if the man is able to move up close inside her, she may feel deep, internal pressure on her G-spot, which will heighten her enjoyment. In addition, her crossed legs put pressure on her thighs, raising the level of pelvic tension, which will assist the build-up of excitement.

From this position, she can use her hands to reach down and stroke her partner's testicles, or reach up and draw her fingertips across his neck and chest. Gentle scratching shows your enjoyment and helps to increase his passion. He may take pleasure from watching her, stroking her body, and from the long, sensuous build-up to climax that this position gives.

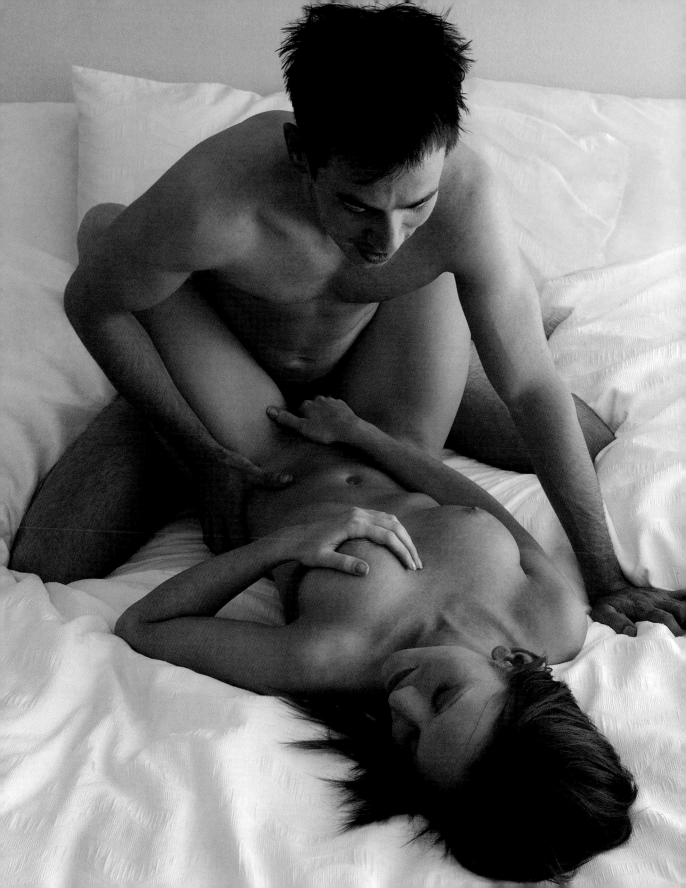

flower in a vase

Extend your lovemaking, and experience all-over-body orgasms

The "climax all over" approach gives men and women the opportunity to experience the sensation of orgasm throughout their whole body. Some lucky women manage this spontaneously, but not many men can.

One of the functional problems with intercourse is that, if a man continues thrusting deeply, then he is likely to reach climax quickly. If a rapid climax is what you both want, then there's no problem. But many men and women feel cheated by having an orgasm before they have fully enjoyed sexual union.

If you want to attain whole-body orgasms, you make love until you are both very close to climax, then rest before going back to pleasuring the whole body again. This method builds sexual excitement and delays orgasm, meaning that the couple has time to fully savor the special rituals that make sex fun.

Flower in a vase begins with the woman lying back and placing her thighs over her man's thighs while he kneels over her to penetrate her. When he feels close to climax, he stops thrusting while his "stalk" remains within her "vase." Ideally, he continues stimulating her by using his fingers while he rests.

Alternatively, the woman can use a mini-vibrator that fits neatly over the finger (see pages 164–165). They run on a tiny battery, and are conveniently unobtrusive.

He can massage her buttocks while she rubs her clitoris. Once he feels in control of his ejaculation, and can see that she is now very aroused indeed, lovers can nudge each other back into action. The benefit of resting in this way is that it can help you to achieve orgasm simultaneously if you so desire.

• SEXUAL MAPPING

The object of this exercise is to discover, through touching your partner's body all over, which parts are sexually responsive. The method involves one partner sitting in the nude while the person doing the "mapping" strokes small areas of his or her partner's skin. These areas should be stroked once or twice with a finger. Work your way down your partner's head, face, neck, shoulders, chest, arms, hands, and so on, right down to their little toes. After each stroke, the partner being stroked rates the eroticism of the touch on a plus three/minus three scale. For example, if strokes on the elbow were uninteresting, they might rate as minus two, while if strokes across the nipple felt especially arousing, these might be scored as plus three.

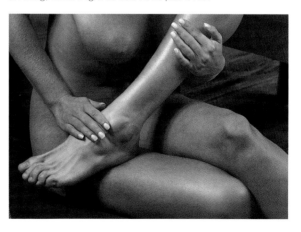

the grip

Use your muscles to squeeze your man to an intense orgasm

Most men love "the grip" because of the increased pressure on the penis as the woman squeezes it between her thighs while he's inside.

Here, the woman lies on her back, and the man lies on top of her. Once his penis is inside her, she brings her legs together underneath him, and squeezes her thighs tightly together while squeezing her vaginal muscles at the same time.

In this position, the man is gripped not just by her vagina but also by her thighs. The sensation for him during thrusting is greatly enhanced because of the greater pressure on his penis. In this position, she will enjoy intense clitoral stimulation as pressing her thighs together bunches her labia up against his penis.

"The grip" is a good position if his erection is not quite hard enough, and it is also helpful for men who take a long time to be stimulated to climax.

• PENIS RING

The medical term for a male erectile problem where the blood flows into the penis during arousal causing an erection, but then flows out again leaving it limp is venous leakage. In such cases, a man can use a medically designed penis ring, available from pharmacists. This clamps around the base of the penis tightly enough to keep the blood flow in, without being dangerous.

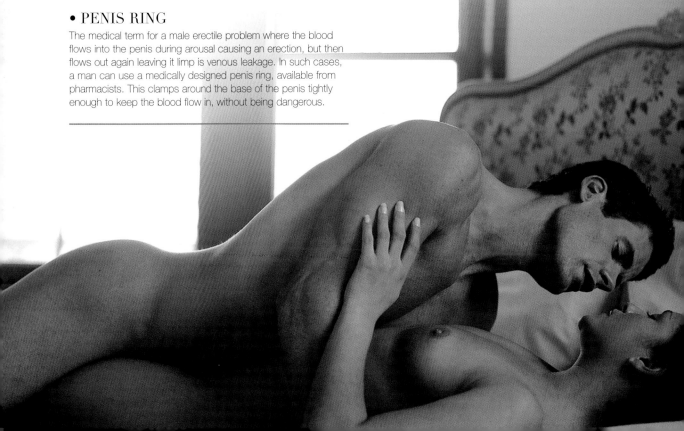

deep penetration

Arouse your woman, then indulge her deepest desires

Even the thought of this erotic position may prove titillating to many women; she will feel stretched wide open during sex, and may gain considerable pleasure from such an intense sexual experience.

Some women enjoy, even need, very deep penetration from sex, perhaps because their cervix or G-spot benefits from internal pressure. This pose offers the woman such deep penetration and pleasure that it can

bring her lover heightened sensitivity. Many men find that sharing the intensity of their lover's arousal brings them to a stronger climax too.

Once she is fully aroused, the man kneels down between her legs, then lifts her left leg up over his right shoulder and tucks her right leg under his left arm. Now he can penetrate and use his hands to caress her. The combination of G-spot pressure and rubbing her clitoris can bring her quickly to orgasm.

• TRIPLE-X FOREPLAY
Spend time stroking, kissing, and licking your woman on the lips, breasts, and genitals before trying this, or any deeply penetrative position. During foreplay, particularly oral sex, the woman's vagina undergoes a process called "tenting," in which the upper end enlarges, so it can accommodate a deep-thrusting penis more comfortably.

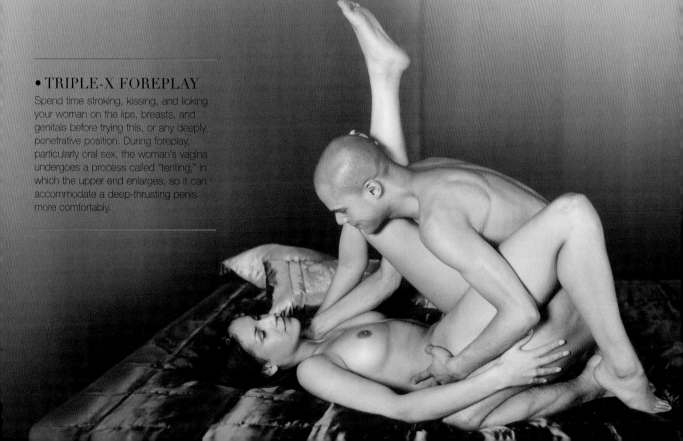

sticky hips

Show him how hot you are for him by sticking to him like glue

This is a tantalizing position for him, as his woman raises up her pelvis to meet his thrusts. He should follow her movements carefully, taking care that his penis does not slip out.

She lies on her back with her knees bent and her feet and shoulders supporting her weight. He leans over her and supports himself on his hands and knees.

She pushes up onto the balls of her feet and lifts her hips to allow him to enter her, then drops her pelvis down suddenly. She continues to lift and drop her pelvis, and he should try and follow her movement,

although it's not entirely easy to do. Don't get too hung up on achieving it: the attraction of this pose is as much the fun that sexual games can bring as the stimulation it offers. When it does work, however, the act of pushing up to meet your man's thrusts can feel sexy and empowering, albeit tiring.

• TEASE WITHOUT TOUCHING

The more something is promised to you, and the longer you have to wait for it, the greater the build-up of anticipation. Tease your lover with the promise of things to come, by exploring all the sexy spots on his or her body. Plant clusters of little kisses behind their knees. Blow kisses in his ears or chew her ear lobes. Finish by sucking your lover's fingers one by one.

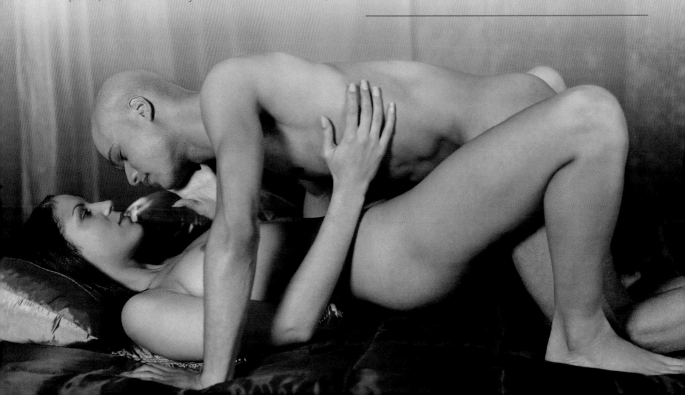

rocking horse

Use a seesaw movement to pleasure your clitoris and G-spot

Women-on-top positions can be very intense for the man, and he may find it difficult not to climax too quickly when faced with the erotic sight, and feel, of her making all the moves on top of him.

This position is helpful in slowing down, or speeding up, the action of lovemaking, and ensures the woman receives enough stimulation on her hot spots to reach a climax at the same time as her man. She leans forward as she slides down on her partner's penis, and tilts her body backward as she rises up. This see-saw movement will hit her most sensitive spots.

By leaning forward and down, the base of his penis is more likely to slide up and along her clitoris, and by tilting backward and rising up, the head of his penis should bump right across her G-spot. Slow rocking also intensifies orgasm for both partners.

• SEXUAL RESPONSE

Men and women experience three main stages of sexual response: desire, arousal, and orgasm. Desire can happen as a result of a look, a touch, or a suggestion. Arousal happens through sexual touch, foreplay, and intercourse. Orgasm happens at the peak of excitement as a happy reflex of whole-body sensuality. After orgasm, the body returns to its resting state.

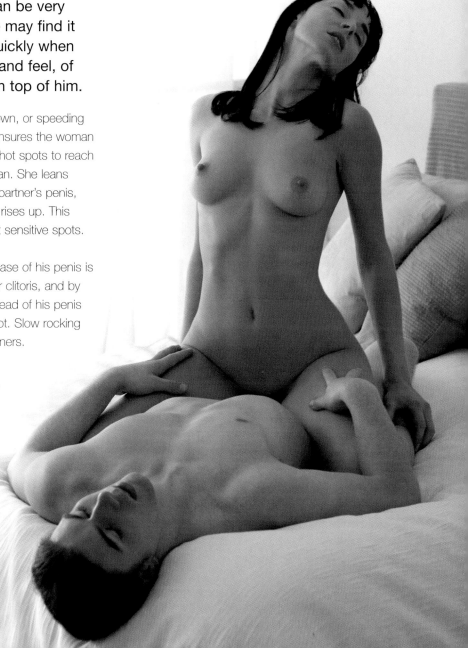

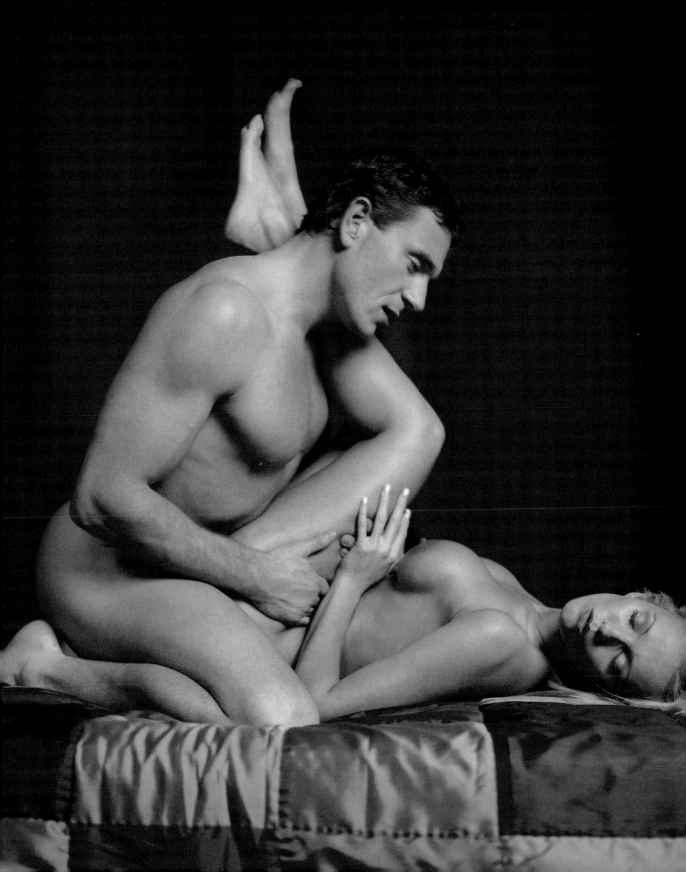

legs sideways

Slow down your orgasm and flex to increase feeling

Positions such as "legs sideways," where penetration is deep and the vagina is squeezed, are excellent for the older man who needs a robust sensation during sex, and satisfying for his woman too.

In this position, the man's penis will feel tightly gripped inside his partner's vagina, while the pressure of his lover's thighs gives him additional friction that may be necessary to bring him to orgasm.

The woman lies back on the bed and raises her legs in the air. Her partner enters her from a kneeling position. He then lifts her legs higher to rest them against his shoulder and begins to thrust.

The woman presses her knees and thighs together to constrict his penis, while clenching and unclenching her vaginal muscles to gain, and give, pleasurable sensations. Her pressed thighs squeeze his penis and her clitoris, helping each partner achieve maximum sensation from his thrusting.

To experience an enhanced orgasm in this position, try using a Tantric sex-training exercise while making love. It is suitable for men and women of all ages and can help both partners to slow down their orgasms, making them last longer and sensationally stronger. It may only take a few practice sessions for couples to significantly extend orgasm time.

During ejaculation the man flexes his penis (see panel below) and the woman contracts her vagina while they both dramatically slow down their thrusting movements. Practiced successfully, this can make a couple's sexual experience so sensual that it is hard to tell when the orgasm begins and ends.

• FLEX TO INCREASE HIS FEELING

Men can use this exercise to increase penile feeling during lovemaking. First of all, the man masturbates to orgasm, and when he ejaculates he counts the contractions of his orgasm. On the next occasion he masturbates again to orgasm, but when he begins to ejaculate he clenches his pelvic floor muscles as he might do if trying to stop the flow of urine. He continues masturbating very slowly while continuing to clench his muscles, pushing himself on through the clenching sensation. If he counts the contractions again during this new experience he will almost certainly find that there are more of them, and the number increases as he practices. Climax is likely to be slighter than normal at the start of the exercises, but more intense by the end.

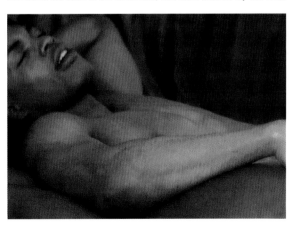

legs raised

Prolong sex and stimulate her G-spot in this satisfying position

This unusual lovemaking position looks fairly acrobatic, but it's easy to get into. The man will like it because his lover is so open to him and he can thrust deeply, but there are hidden benefits for her too.

The woman lies back, opens her legs, and then places her feet on her partner's chest. He kneels close to her to penetrate. In this position, he will probably find it harder to get highly aroused, which is useful if she wants the action to last a little longer.

The other advantage of this pose is that it makes G-spot stimulation easier. Regular thrusting doesn't normally provide the intense and localized pressure necessary to stimulate the G-spot, but here he can lean back so that his penis is pressed against the uppermost side of her vagina where the G-spot lies.

Women: to make this position a visual and physical treat for your man, clench your muscles and give a little wiggle from time to time. The sight and sensation of you will prove orgasmic for him.

• G-SPOT ORGASM

When a woman experiences sustained pressure on her G-spot (see page 36), it can trigger an orgasm. In fact, some women who have G-spot orgasms also ejaculate a thin arc of fluid when climaxing in this way. To stimulate your G-spot, exert a steady pressure with your finger, pushing on it for a count of 10, then let go, then press again. Remember it is pressure not light stroking that stimulates this orgasmic center.

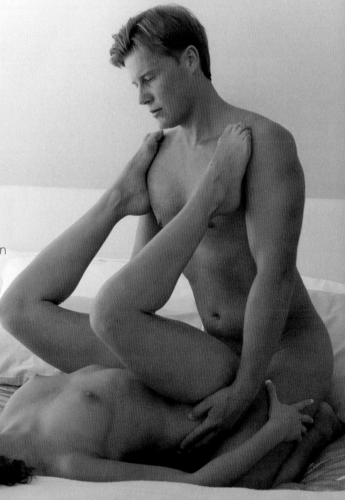

widely open

Surrender yourself to your man by opening your legs wide

Many women instinctively open their legs wide for penetration and, with this sexy gesture, offer themselves to a lover. Being nestled between his woman's legs is a powerful turn-on for any man.

Here, the woman lies back, lifts her legs, and opens her thighs widely. This enables her man to place his knees on either side of her hips, and lean gently against her to thrust and grind.

The couple can choose to hold onto each other, or the man can use his free hands to massage her breasts and stroke her abdomen.

Although this position feels erotic, it may not provide either lover with very much sensation. The barrier of her uplifted thighs doesn't allow for deep penetration, so her clitoris does not receive much stimulation. However, the undeniable eroticism and helplessness you feel in this position will be exciting, and a sensual precursor to more robust lovemaking positions.

• THE PULSAR TECHNIQUE

The pulsar technique enhances the sensation of orgasm in the man. It can be used by either partner, but should be done during ejaculation. Masturbate your partner to orgasm. As he climaxes, clasp your hands around the head of your man's penis. Squeeze gently, hold for a second, then let go. Pause. Then do it again. The trick is to time your pulsations with his contractions.

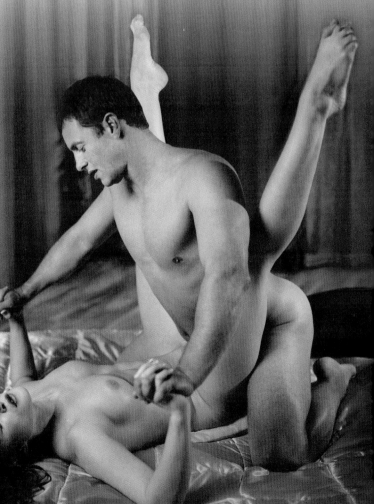

erotic strokes

Erotic stroking consists of just about everything that can please the body, with one exception—sexual intercourse. The benefit of stroking is that it enables couples to get to know each other's bodies in great detail. Couples learn which areas of the body respond to touch, and how to pace lovemaking so that each partner grows more and more excited. Above all, erotic stroking encourages couples to explore the notion of "delayed gratification" because there is no pressure to make each other climax.

Light caresses

Start by having a long soak in a warm bath together. Next give each other an all-over massage using sweet-smelling oils. Take turns stroking each other's bodies.

As you touch your lover's body, and are touched, note the erotic sensations that grow beneath your fingers. Focus particularly on the abdomen, thighs, buttocks, chest, nipples, lower legs, and feet. If certain areas feel more sensual than others, build on the enjoyable feelings there. Avoid touching the genitals for now.

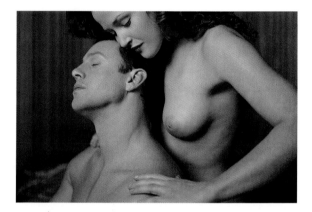

Ensure your hands are well-lubricated with massage oil before you starting stroking each other, to ensure that they slip easily across each other's responsive skin.

Stroking the chest

Some women (but not all) have incredibly sensitive breasts. To find out her response, lightly oil and manipulate her breasts, making sure that you pay particular attention to the nipples and areolae.

Similarly, for many (but not all) men, the nipples are a rich source of eroticism. Stroking, touching, tweaking, or tickling the nipples will create prickles of sensation and anticipation that flood through many other parts of his body, and can result in a erection.

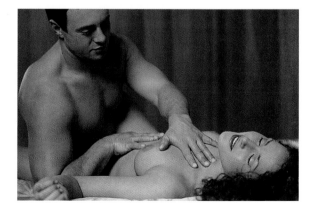

Use a light circling stroke across the chest. Start at the shoulders and stroke down the torso. Move the breasts in circles, and trace your fingertips around the nipples.

Stroking the genitals

Once you have stroked and caressed each other's bodies thoroughly, you are ready to move on to your partner's genitals.

Men: massage and stroke her labia, clitoris, and vagina. Concentrate on the strokes and the areas that your woman responds positively to. Most women prefer a light touch on the genitals, although everyone differs in the kind of pressure they prefer.

Locate the area on the entrance to the vagina that gives the best sensation. If direct contact with the clitoris feels too strong, she may find it more pleasurable to be caressed through a silk scarf or choose to use one of the many vibrators that are available (see pages 164–165).

Women: gently fondle his penis. If he is not circumcised, ease his foreskin away from the tip on each downward stroke. Try shaking the penis a little, or simply rubbing round or over it. You may want to use lubrication to ensure comfort, particularly if he is circumcised.

As his penis stiffens, slip your hand right down the shaft, then back up again. Repeat this several times. If your man is uncircumcised, do this by moving the foreskin up and down. As his erection becomes hard, focus on stimulating the head. Grasp the penis on the ridge that encircles the tip, and move the skin backward and forward. Sensation here can be especially dynamic, and some men like climaxing from this kind of movement alone.

....

Work your way slowly across your partner's stomach, buttocks, and thighs to touch their genitals, Make them feel that you have all the time in the world.

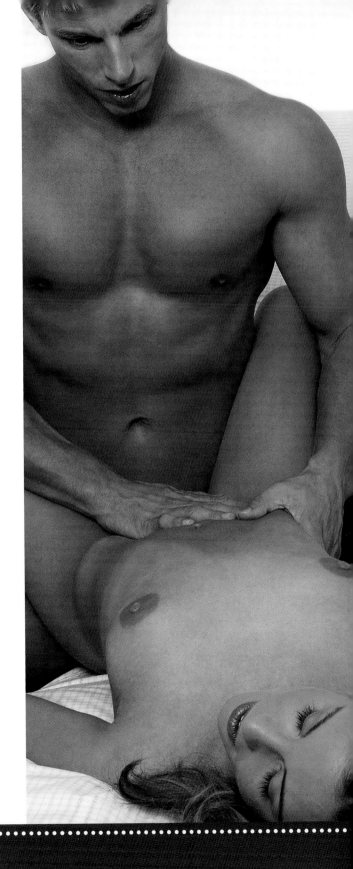

steady pressure

Increase orgasmic friction with plenty of close contact

Friction is essential for sexual stimulation. Some positions, such as this one, offer particularly close, intense contact, which uses rhythmic pressure and clitoral stimulation to excite her.

The woman lies on her front but rolls slightly on her side and props herself up with one arm. He enters her from behind, and pushes and circles his penis inside her vagina to keep prolonged pressure on her G-spot (see page 36). He also places his hand between her legs and uses the "seizure" technique. This involves manipulating the top of her pubic mound to expose her clitoris while he penetrates her, so that he presses it against the shaft of his penis.

• STRENGTHENING EXERCISES

Use these simple exercises to strengthen your vaginal muscles, and improve your sexual performance. Start by squeezing your vagina tight then relaxing, as often as you can. After a week of practising, try "fluttering" your muscles—squeezing and relaxing in quick succession. A week later, add the "hydraulic elevator" to your repertoire. Imagine the interior of your vagina is an elevator shaft. Squeeze your vagina closed in order to get the elevator up to the first floor, then move on to the second floor, and so on until you reach the top. Here, squeeze again then repeat the sequence until you reach the bottom.

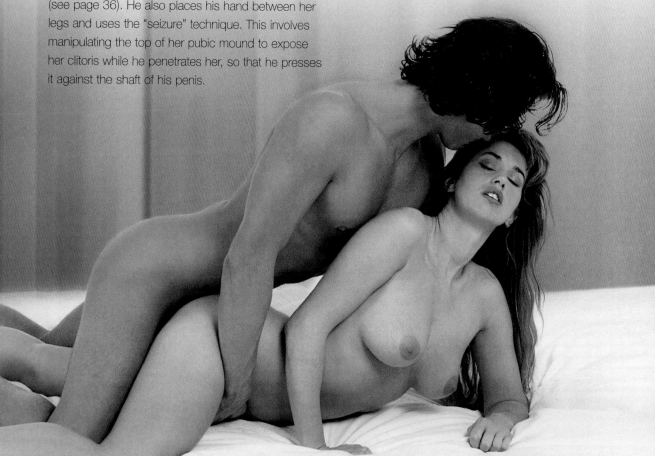

the press

Curl up beneath his body, and submit to his desires

In this position, the woman draws her legs up and places both feet together on her partner's chest to achieve an erotic and submissive pose.

With his lover offering such complete surrender, he will feel very aroused by her vulnerability and his own powerful strength. He can gently hold onto one of her knees to help him thrust. But, like the "leg stretch" position (see page 105), he must be careful not to thrust too hard into his lover's shortened vagina.

Having the woman's feet flat on his chest is likely to increase the intensity of the man's feelings. It can be a surprisingly loving gesture should he choose to caress her foot, possibly even raising it to kiss her toes or caress her ankle as a demonstration of affection.

For the woman, lying in this defenseless position may bring erotic, subconscious feelings to the surface while you make love. Caress his thighs in rhythm with his thrusting movements to enhance his enjoyment.

• SWEET-SMELLING SKIN
All humans smell, although not necessarily unpleasant. In the best circumstances it can be a pure aphrodisiac. The strength of body scent depends largely on diet. If you change from a spicy, diet to a vegetarian, unspiced, or herbal diet, you will find that your body odor sweetens too.

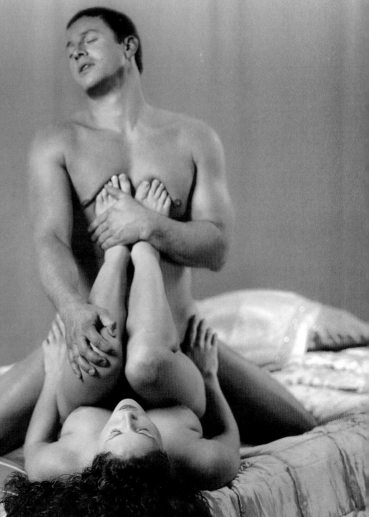

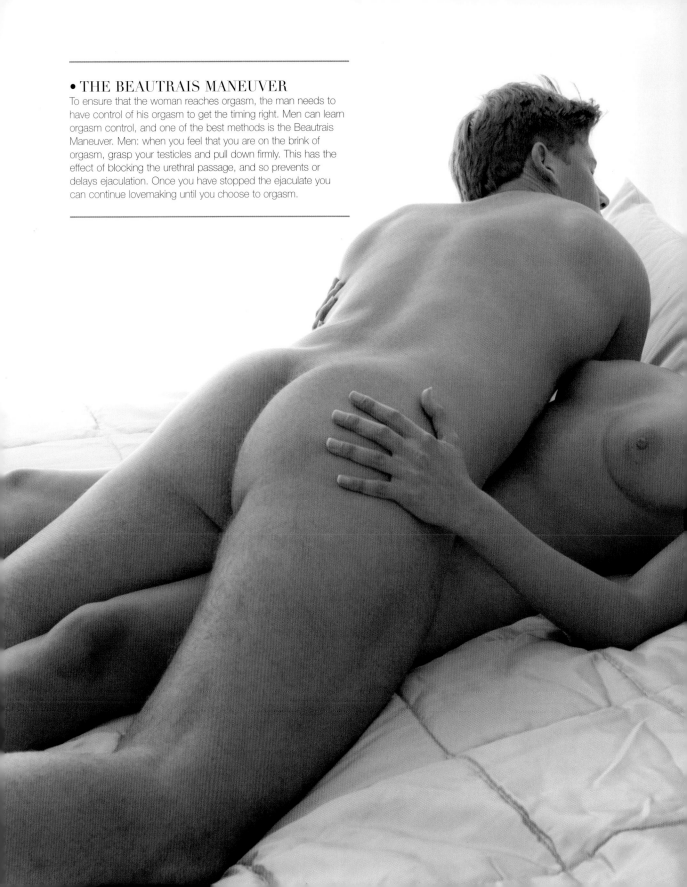

• THE BEAUTRAIS MANEUVER

To ensure that the woman reaches orgasm, the man needs to have control of his orgasm to get the timing right. Men can learn orgasm control, and one of the best methods is the Beautrais Maneuver. Men: when you feel that you are on the brink of orgasm, grasp your testicles and pull down firmly. This has the effect of blocking the urethral passage, and so prevents or delays ejaculation. Once you have stopped the ejaculate you can continue lovemaking until you choose to orgasm.

scissors

Let your excitement mount slowly into an explosive orgasm

In any sexual position, the build-up of sexual excitement and tension is vital. Orgasm is the relief of this sexual tension. It can be difficult, and sometimes impossible, to achieve climax if tension is not allowed to build.

This position allows for maximum pressure on both the male and female pubic areas. Seen from above, the couple make a kind of scissor shape. The woman lies on her back and her man is on top. But instead of lying stretched out along her body, he lies with one of his legs between hers. This alters the angle of the top half of his body so that, although his and her abdomens are touching, the man is actually lying to one side of her. This means that his arms are bearing some of the weight, and he is not crushing his partner.

As you make love, your two pelvises act like a kind of fulcrum, rocking backward and forward on each other as he thrusts. The areas around the pelvis, in particular the thighs and buttocks, become a focus of sexual tension. It is possible to aid and enhance climax by building up muscles in these areas by exercises such as running. In addition, men and women can practice bio-energetic exercises, such as flexing the thighs and buttocks, or Kegel exercises, both of which assist couples in achieving heightened orgasms.

sensuous paddle

Reach a satisfying climax with an in-out, rocking motion

The twin movements of penetration and withdrawal in this position are slow and erotic, and mimic the languid dog-paddle motion of a turtle afloat in tropical seas.

In this position, the woman lies on her back with her legs raised and bent toward her chest. He kneels up, holds onto her uplifted thighs, and thrusts into her with slow and deliberate moves.

The man should pull his penis out almost entirely before commencing each following stroke. As her man does this, the woman pulls back from his penis to feel the long withdrawal, then pushes forward as he slowly penetrates her again.

The slow, deliberate movements of lovemaking can be very exciting, especially combined with his tight hold on her legs. This and the resistance of their bodies against each other can lead both partners to orgasm.

• "NOTHING" SESSION
Time spent doing nothing allows lovers to experience eroticism without physical contact. Find a quiet room and set a timer for 30 minutes. Lie facing your lover, with or without clothes, and look into each other's eyes. Allow yourself to enter a trance-like state and go with your feelings. When the timer sounds, end your reverie with a kiss then share your thoughts.

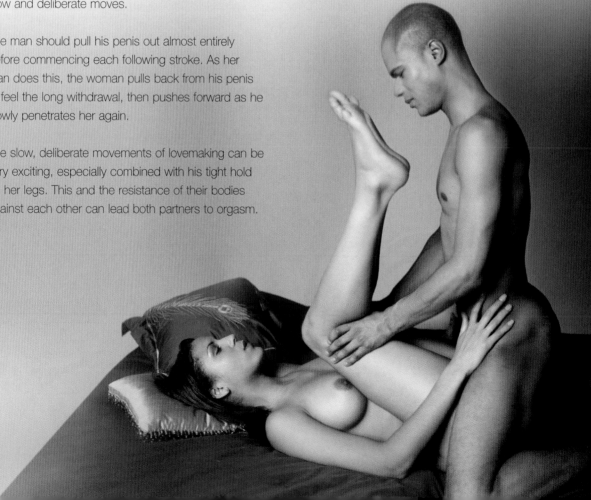

g-spot bliss

Indulge in deep penetration and G-spot stimulation

Positions in which the woman lies on her back as the man kneels to enter her allow the man to dominate sex. She enjoys an erotic sense of helplessness, and he is able to penetrate deeply.

The woman lies on her back and bends her legs at the knees to draw them back as close as she can to her chest. Her man kneels with his knees either side of her buttocks, and moves into the most comfortable position to penetrate her.

She can gain pleasure by holding onto her knees and raising her hips higher, so that her partner can penetrate her more deeply and at an angle in which his penis stimulates her highly sensitive G-spot. The G-spot is on the upper wall of the vagina, so specially angled thrusting is required to reach it.

Men: if you are hoping to give your woman a G-spot orgasm, remember that it is sustained pressure on the spot rather than the friction of thrusting that provides the necessary stimulation.

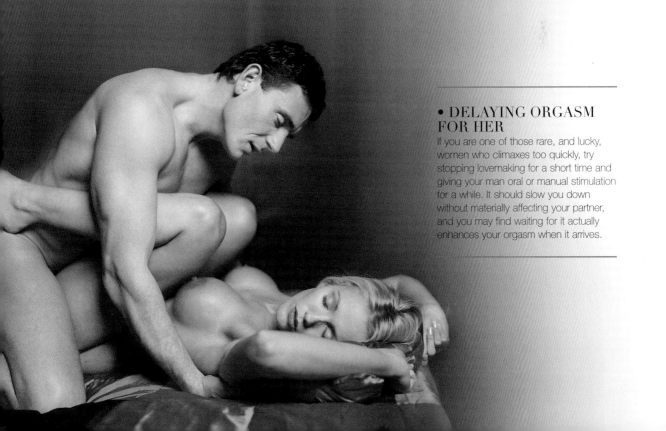

• DELAYING ORGASM FOR HER

If you are one of those rare, and lucky, women who climaxes too quickly, try stopping lovemaking for a short time and giving your man oral or manual stimulation for a while. It should slow you down without materially affecting your partner, and you may find waiting for it actually enhances your orgasm when it arrives.

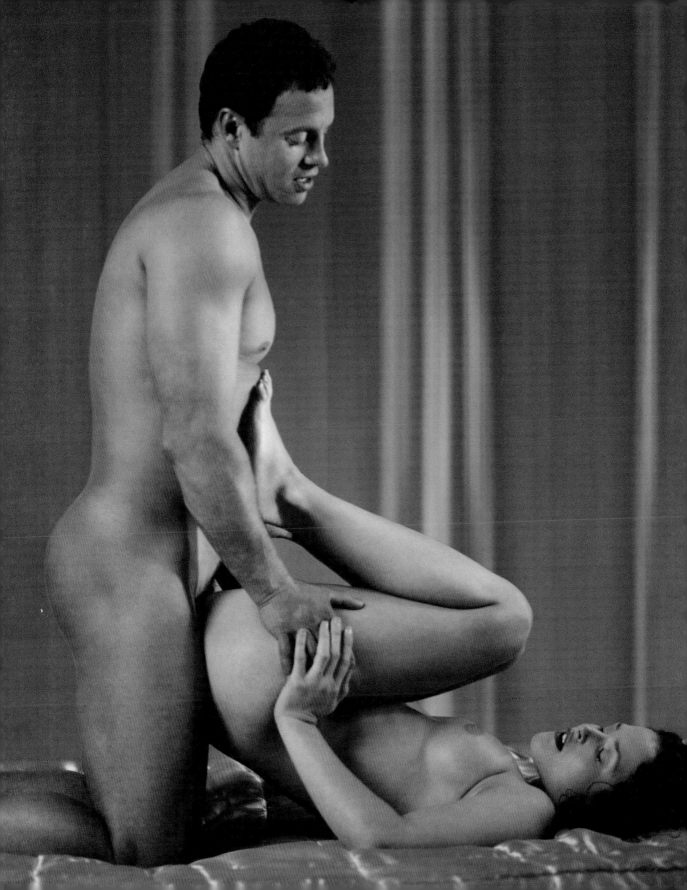

the temptress

Spice up your love life with this pleasurable and exotic position

This position allows for lovemaking in which the woman's vagina is fully open, and allows the man to attain maximum penetration while putting pressure on the woman's sensitive G-spot and cervix.

Here, the woman bends her knees and draws them up to her body. The man lifts her hips to penetrate her while holding onto her thighs to control his thrusts.

This is a supremely comfortable kneeling sex position for the man if his weight and height are compatible with his partner's. If their bodies align well, he can lean against her and thrust without straining his arms or legs. She can achieve considerable arousal by tensing her vaginal muscles when the knees are bent and drawn up in this way. Her partner can also use his hands to stroke her clitoris and perineum.

The combination of sensations causes a deep sexual tension to build up in the pelvic area, especially in the thighs and buttocks. As pleasure peaks, this mounting tension explodes into orgasm. For the woman, the tension can be intensified if she finds herself excited by being bundled up into a package.

Your man may find it hard to resist you in this position, but it is possible to delay his orgasm by pressing on his Jen-Mo point. This is a Taoist method of preventing ejaculation. Pressing hard on the Jen-Mo point—a pressure point halfway between the anus and the scrotum—constricts the flow of ejaculate. However, you need to be accurate about where you press. If you apply pressure too close to the anus it won't work, but if you press too close to the scrotum, his semen will go into his bladder, making his urine cloudy.

• SEX OUT LOUD

It's often said that the most important sex organ is the brain. Sharing erotic ideas that engage the imagination will give you both a sense of playful enjoyment. Titillating your man with erotic ideas and suggestions is a powerful means of seduction. The secret is to describe in very precise detail exactly what you are going to do to your lover. For example, tell him that you're going to kiss him along the length of his spine, then you're going to turn him over so that you can kiss and stroke his penis. Finally, you're going to climb on top and slide yourself on to his erect penis. The sexiest way to deliver these kinds of suggestions is by whispering them in your lover's ear. When you've completed your description, make sure you deliver what you have promised.

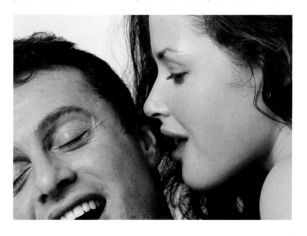

tails entwined

Get close to each other for an exciting new angle of penetration

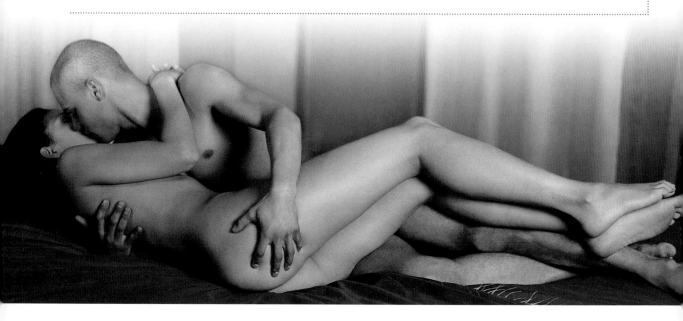

The arrangement of lovers' legs in this position resembles two fishes bending their tails around each others' bodies as they writhe together to mate.

The couple lie side-by-side facing each other, with their legs stretched out. After penetration, the man lifts the woman's legs—which she holds together—and places them on top of his own.

This is a good position for shallow, sensitive strokes. The man can alter the angle of penetration by moving his lover's legs slightly. The lovers then undulate together rhythmically until they reach climax. For this

kind of front-on, side-by-side sex to work well, the man needs quite a long penis since, due to the position of her legs, he can only penetrate a short way.

This position is perfect after an all-over massage when both of your bodies are slick with massage oil, and lovemaking can be slow, leisurely, and slippery.

• MASTURBATION
Mutual masturbation is a key ingredient of lovemaking. Manual sex ensures she achieves maximum pleasure, and gives a break from the intensity of penetration. It works particularly well with sex positions such as "tails entwined" which don't allow for much stimulation of the clitoris during sex. Share your favorite strokes with each other to know how to best pleasure each other.

---

pressed thighs

Heighten your **sexual awareness** in this erotically visual position

Exchanging eye contact while stroking each others' legs adds to the emotional and physical intensity of this comfortable, but satisfying sitting position.

Save this one for making love in front of the fire, or in the bath when you just can't contain your passion. Or you might find this position evolves naturally from sitting and cuddling your lover.

The woman lowers herself down onto the man's penis as he sits with his legs wide apart. Once he has penetrated her fully, he presses her thighs tightly together with his hands while he thrusts into her.

He can increase the pleasurable sensations of his penis being squeezed by his woman's constricted vagina if he keeps her thighs pressed tightly together.

As she leans back on her elbows the couple can gaze into each others' faces, and watch each other's mounting excitement as they strive toward orgasm.

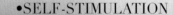

•SELF-STIMULATION
Most women love the closeness and fullness they experience during sex in a sitting position. However, they may not necessarily enjoy intense climaxes this way. Women: it is a good idea to practice self-stimulation so that you learn your own orgasmic patterns as well as your erogenous zones. If you know what turns you on, then you can take this information into your sexual relationship.

oral stimulation

Many people enjoy the sensations and intimacy of oral sex. Fellatio is done to the man, and consists of the manipulation of the penis by mouth. The man may climax in his partner's mouth, or she may prefer to substitute a hand or tissue for the last stage of the proceedings. Cunnilingus is performed on the woman, and involves manipulation of the clitoris by the man's tongue. Every woman's clitoral sensitivity differs; ask her occasionally for feedback. Simultaneous oral sex is known as "69" (see pages 84–85).

Licking the penis

Start by treating his penis like an ice-cream cone, holding it at the base and licking all over, running your tongue slowly up and down the shaft. Then take the penis into your mouth and slide your lips gradually down to its base (or about halfway) and back again.

Alternatively, experiment with fellating the head only (the most sensitive area of a man's penis), including hand stimulation at the same time. Suck vigorously or move his penis around your mouth as if brushing your teeth with it.

Fellatio techniques

With his penis in your hand, kiss it gently as though you were kissing his lower lip. Next, twirl your tongue around the penis head, taking care to rub across the coronal ridge and the frenulum – usually the most sensitive spots.

Hold his penis between your fingers, then kiss and delicately nibble the sides. You could also try out the butterfly flick. Hold the base of his penis and take the head in your mouth. As your mouth moves up and down, flicker your tongue rapidly back and forward across the frenulum.

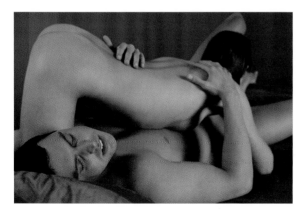

Find a comfortable position, such as this top-to-tail pose, which gives you maximum access and means he can stroke your clitoris with his fingers at the same time.

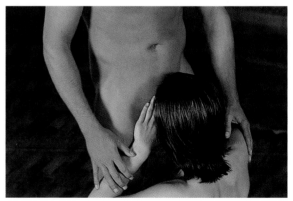

Extend your mouth by making a ring around the top of his penis using your thumb and fingers, then keep the "ring" against your mouth as you move up and down.

Cunnilingus

The clitoris is probably the most sensitive zone of a woman's body. For cunnilingus to work well, you should position yourself between your woman's legs so that you can cover her clitoris and labia with the broad blade of your tongue.

Position your head between, and slightly below her thighs so that you can stroke your tongue upward over the shaft and head of her clitoris, then stimulate each side of the clitoris in turn, always working from the base to the top.

Experiment with your tongue tip and blade. Try stimulating one side of the clitoris, then the other. Occasionally ring your tongue around her vaginal entrance, and insert your tongue inside.

Feather-light tongue-twirling on top of the clitoris itself can be sensational. Try this in a clockwise, then counterclockwise direction, then flick the tip of the tongue from side to side immediately beneath it the clitoris. Try covering the clitoris with your mouth gently and flicking your tongue firmly across it at the same time.

Run your tongue along and between her labia and insert your tongue into her vagina, moving your tongue up and down and in and out, using both shallow and deep strokes. Lightly lick up and down her perineum—the area between the vagina and anus—using the tip of your tongue.

The secret to good cunnilingus is to focus on the place where she most enjoys stimulation, and not to move around too much.

....

Position yourself so that you are comfortable, and can stimulate the clitoris from underneath. Be very gentle as this area is extremely sensitive and can bruise easily.

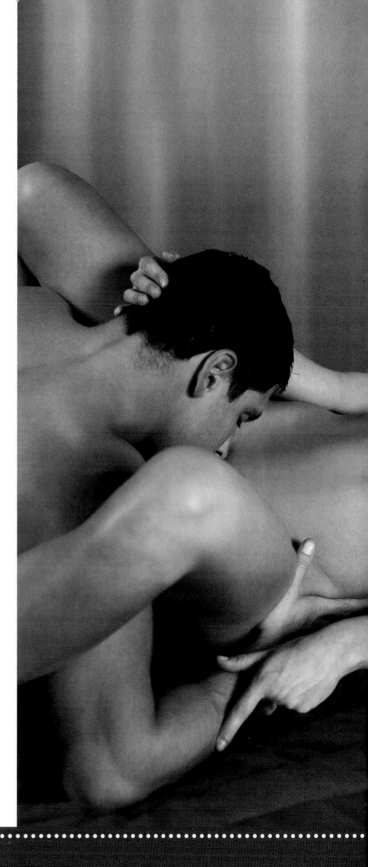

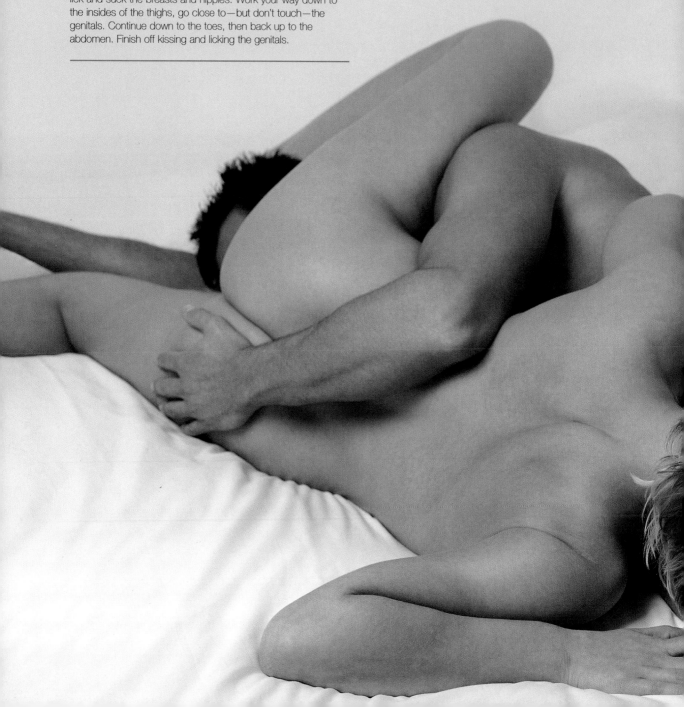

• TONGUE BATHING

Tongue bathing should only be done in a luxuriously warm room. Before you begin, share a sensual bath or shower together. Towel each other off, and begin your oral exploration of your partner's body. Start by kissing and licking his or her mouth and face. Work your way slowly around the ears and down the neck and throat to the shoulders. When you move on to the chest, lick and suck the breasts and nipples. Work your way down to the insides of the thighs, go close to—but don't touch—the genitals. Continue down to the toes, then back up to the abdomen. Finish off kissing and licking the genitals.

soixante-neuf

Move into this delectable pose for intense, mutual oral pleasure

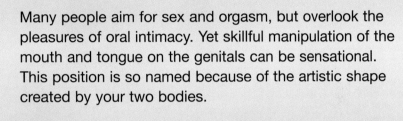

Many people aim for sex and orgasm, but overlook the pleasures of oral intimacy. Yet skillful manipulation of the mouth and tongue on the genitals can be sensational. This position is so named because of the artistic shape created by your two bodies.

The "69" position allows you snuggle up to each other, head to genitals, and give each other oral sex at the same time. Simultaneous oral sex requires a large degree of trust. And, as a result, it can be a deeply satisfying experience for both partners.

However, some people prefer receiving oral sex separately (see pages 82–83), on the grounds that if they focus entirely on themselves rather than on their partner their sexual sensation will be more intense; equally, if they are performing oral sex on their partner, they can concentrate solely on giving optimum pleasure. If you are unsure about oral sex, it is a good idea to experiment with tongue bathing first (see left).

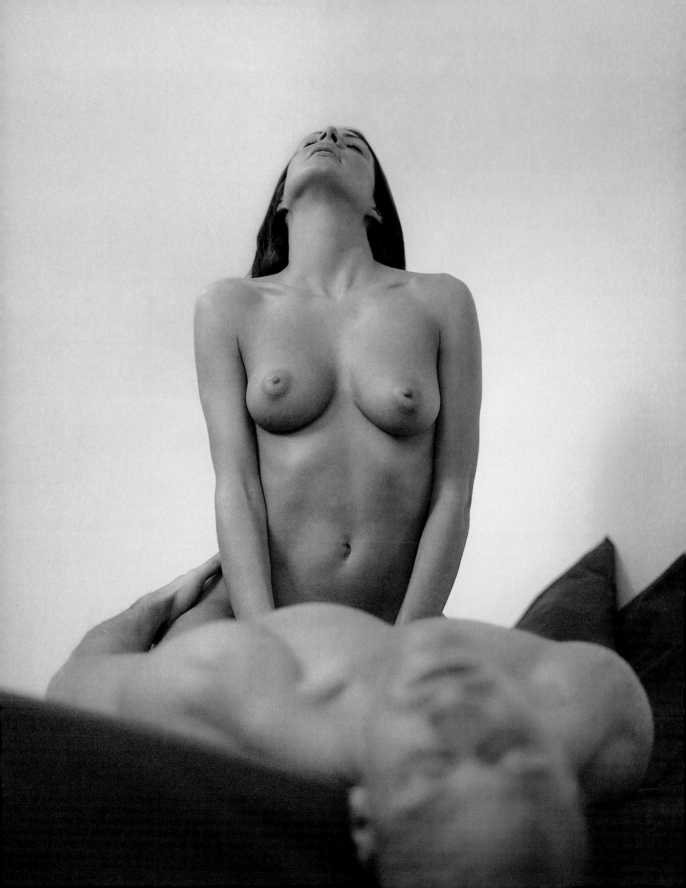

sitting upright

Straddling your man is erotic and sexy, and shows him how hot you are for him. Being on top means the woman takes control of her own arousal, and can set the movement, tempo, and depth of sex.

Here, the woman has her knees bent, facing her man as she sits astride him while he reclines on the bed. She draws his penis slowly into her, and repeatedly squeezes it with her vaginal muscles, holding it tight for a long time. Keeping her back upright means that penetration in this position is deep. And, if she enjoys stimulation on her cervix, she can position herself to attain vigorous, or gentle, sensations inside her.

She can also experiment with the angle of thrusting so that her clitoris is in the direct line of fire to achieve optimum pleasure. She can move forward and backward, as well as sliding up and down his penis. Drawing him slowly up inside her vagina, and stopping just before his penis slips out, to squeeze the head can be intensely exciting for him. And changing the pace of movements from fast to slow will help to maintain excitement for both lovers.

By sitting astride her man, the woman can stimulate herself as well as him. If he doesn't wish to be totally passive, he can use his hands to stroke her or use his fingers to stimulate her clitoris, or reach around to rim a well-lubricated finger around her anus.

This is the perfect method if she wants to initiate sex with her man, as she can slide on top of the erect penis she has just coaxed into life. Alternatively, the man can start off on top then the couple can roll over, reversing their positions. You can wriggle and roll and end up halfway across the room, taking turns on top.

• SECRET STROKES

This technique is for men and women who want to experience their orgasms more fully. During lovemaking, the man alternates the speed of his thrusts, moving his pelvis in time with the ballroom dance rhythm "slow, slow, quick-quick, slow." The technique can feel artificial at first, but the rhythm is so simple that most men soon forget about keeping time, and let it happen naturally. The variation between fast and slow thrusting not only adds variety to both partner's sensations, it also helps the man to reign in his pleasure and delay his orgasm. Women can also use this technique to great effect when in a controlling position such as "sitting upright." By varying the speed and depth of penetration, she can control his arousal.

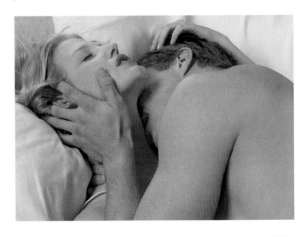

leaning forward

Invite him to play with this sexy woman-on-top pose

"Leaning forward" is a good position for sexually arousing a man if he is feeling weary, or for encouraging him to get in the mood for sex.

The woman can slide playfully on top of him, stroking his chest and genitals with her hands and sensually rubbing her body against his. If she has long hair, she can sweep it across his chest and genitals, and move sensuously down his body, kissing and nibbling him.

Having teased him into an erection, she can mount him from above, tightening her vagina around his penis as she sits down, then lean forward to gently gyrate and rock on top of him.

Stopping to wiggle your hips from time to time will send bolts of excitement through his body, and is a fun way to tease and pleasure him. Men love sexual attention that is focused solely on them, and you can delight him by deciding to make it "his turn."

• MAGIC STROKES
Give him some extra stimulation when you are on top. Some men love their testicles being stroked and handled during intercourse. If you want to give him additional stimulation, keep a finger on the base of his penis or grasp it between your finger and thumb to put additional pressure on it as you move sensuously on top of him.

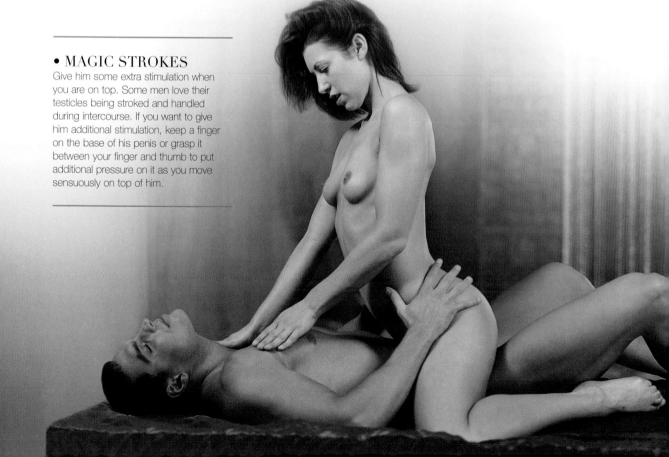

leaning backward

Sit astride your lover and rock yourself to orgasm

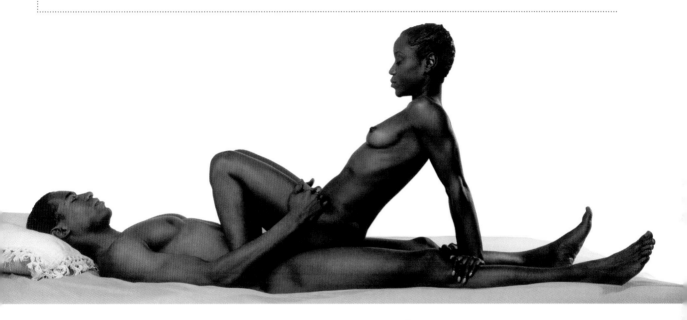

Women-on-top positions are perfect for allowing couples to prolong lovemaking, and experience a range of different sensations without interrupting the flow of sex or the build-up of excitement.

Here, the woman slows the pace and intensity of sex. She leans back and supports her weight on her hands to change the stimulation on his penis. She can lean backward or forward to enjoy shallower strokes, or upright to move his penis in and out of her vagina.

The couple can kiss and stroke each other's bodies as excitement mounts between them, leading their lovemaking to a thrilling climax.

In this lying, hands-free position, the man can also choose to use his fingers to masturbate her during penetration. Masturbation is a key ingredient of lovemaking. Many women find it difficult or even impossible to climax from intercourse alone, so masturbation is an ideal way of ensuring that she achieves maximum pleasure from lovemaking.

• SKIN SENSATIONS

Never underestimate the power of continuing to stroke and kiss your partner during sex. Think of your lover's skin as their biggest sex organ of all. Underneath it lie thousands of nerve endings that send sensational signals to the brain when stimulated. It's entirely through the nerve connections between skin and brain that we get turned on—physically and emotionally.

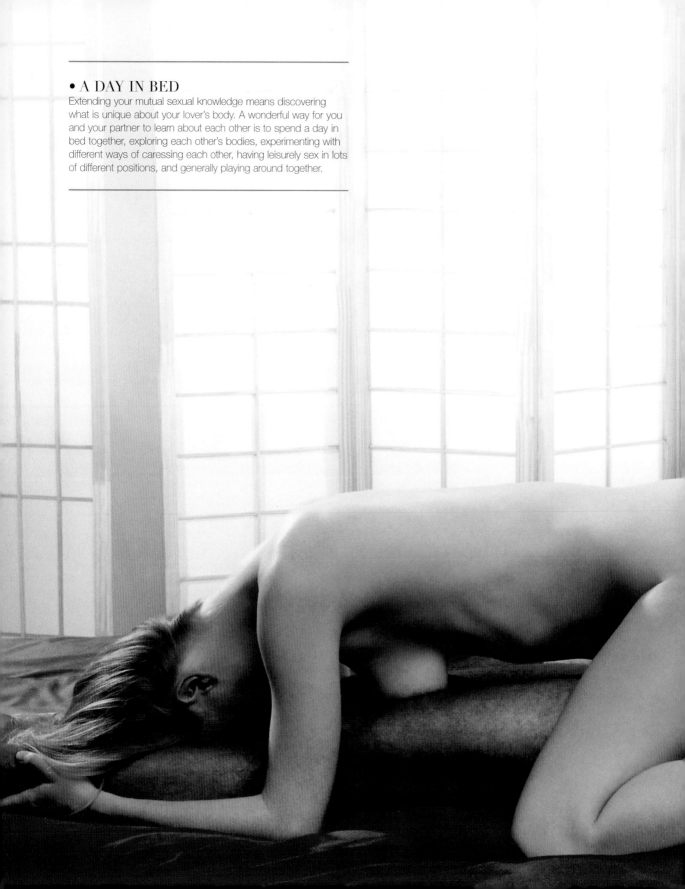

• A DAY IN BED

Extending your mutual sexual knowledge means discovering what is unique about your lover's body. A wonderful way for you and your partner to learn about each other is to spend a day in bed together, exploring each other's bodies, experimenting with different ways of caressing each other, having leisurely sex in lots of different positions, and generally playing around together.

the swing

Try this stretching, swinging position just for the fun of it

If you think the goal of sex is to have an orgasm, you are missing out on most of the fun. Some of the best sex takes place when two people are both just enjoying each others' bodies, and experimenting with new sensations.

In this uncomplicated woman-on-top position, she sits with her back to the man and swings forward and backward, and so consecutively covers and uncovers his penis as she moves. The swinging movements of her vagina across the head of his penis are especially sensual for him, and he can stroke her bottom and watch her move on top of him for extra thrills.

She needs to judge how far forward she can swing before his penis slips out of her vagina. This position makes her partner feel wonderful but has less to offer her by way of stimulation, although she may be aroused by the repeated friction of the penis moving in and out of her vagina.

the voyeur

Gaze upon your lover's body in this stimulating position

Men favor this position because it offers them an erotically titillating view of their partner's labia and body. Watching his penis entering and withdrawing from her vagina will be intensely exciting for him.

This is actually a surprisingly comfortable position for the woman, despite appearances, and has erotic advantages, too. Her pelvic area is relatively unimpeded, giving her easy access to stroke her clitoris should she wish to bring herself to orgasm.

The woman lies on her back, raises her legs up high, and rests them on her partner's shoulders. The man kneels to lift her up gently by the hips, drawing her onto his penis. He makes shallow thrusts to begin with, but gradually, as the vagina becomes moist and she becomes more aroused, his thrusting can grow deeper and stronger.

He can enhance her sexual arousal by describing his mounting excitement and the view, as he watches their erotic coupling from above.

• GETTING DEEPER
If the woman wants to gain deeper penetration in this position she can hold onto her man's shoulders to help push herself onto his penis. The accessibility of her vagina means that the man doesn't have to support his own weight, making it an ideal position for the older or heavier man and his lighter partner.

cross-legged

Help him to orgasm by teasing him from on top

This method is useful for men who suffer from initial erectile problems, or if a woman wishes to continue lovemaking after her man has climaxed.

It is possible to tease a soft penis into the vagina, offering an appreciated starting point for the man, or the possibility of another orgasm for her—provided he wants to continue lovemaking.

The woman sits cross-legged on her man's thighs, and inserts his penis into her vagina. She then moves up and down. By altering the angle of his penis inside her the woman gives herself the stimulation she needs to become highly aroused. This could be either clitoral stimulation from his penis, or from her own fingers as she rises and falls above him. The position has the added bonus of being able to control, to some extent, the contact between his penis and her G-spot.

• STRONGER ORGASMS FOR HIM

Men can develop muscle control to achieve stronger, or even sequential, orgasms. Climax is triggered by muscular tension in the pelvic area. If a man wants to build up these muscles, he can practice this simple exercise while masturbating or being stimulated. Alternately flex and relax your thighs and lower abdomen for as long as possible. Five minutes is the aim, but stop if you get cramp. Excite yourself slowly, building up to a high pitch of arousal. When you are about to reach orgasm, clench your pelvic-floor muscles.

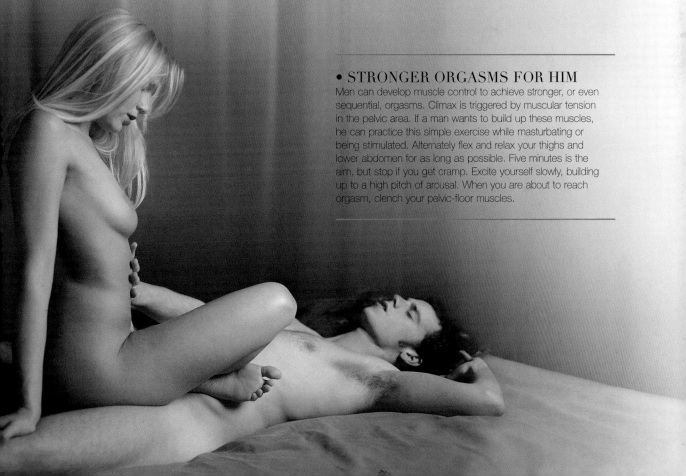

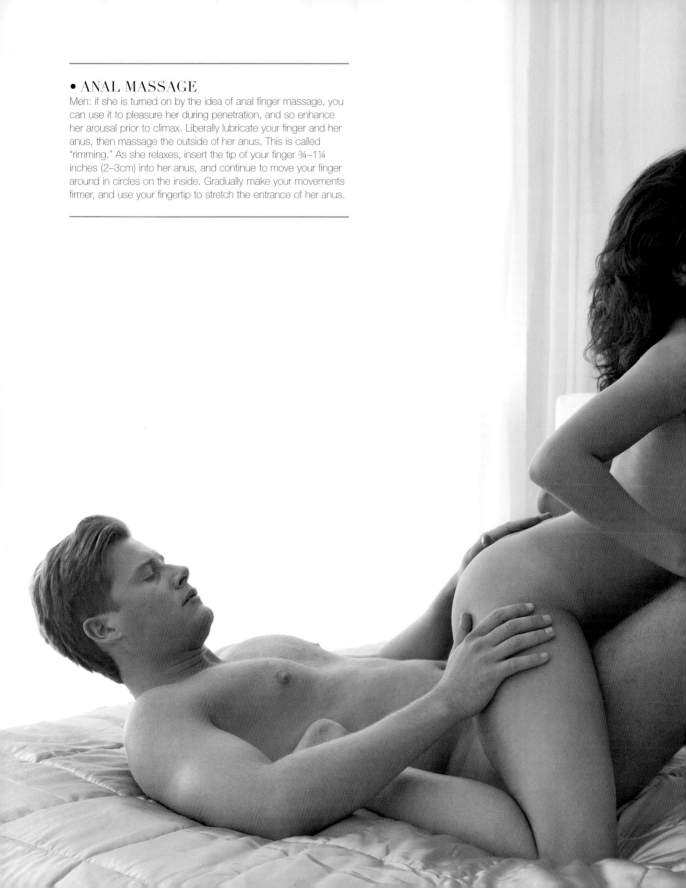

• ANAL MASSAGE

Men: if she is turned on by the idea of anal finger massage, you can use it to pleasure her during penetration, and so enhance her arousal prior to climax. Liberally lubricate your finger and her anus, then massage the outside of her anus. This is called "rimming." As she relaxes, insert the tip of your finger ¾–1¼ inches (2–3cm) into her anus, and continue to move your finger around in circles on the inside. Gradually make your movements firmer, and use your fingertip to stretch the entrance of her anus.

lift and support

Recline and appreciate the view of your woman from behind

Men are generally enthusiastic about women-on-top positions, because they get to relax while their partners take control. This position has extra appeal to him because he also gets a first-rate view of her behind.

The woman sits astride her man backward while he lies on his back with his knees raised. As she rises and falls on his penis, he can support her with his knees to aid her movement. Her balance is best maintained by leaning forward slightly. She can slow down her movements to delay his orgasm; prolonging arousal in this way can allow a greater climax.

Be careful to avoid sudden movements because the unusual angle of intercourse might cause the penis to slip and catch, which can be painful. To give him some extra attention, she can slip a hand between his legs and gently stroke his testicles and perineum.

She may enjoy the sheer eroticism of this position, but it is really his treat as it is difficult for her to receive any extra clitoral stimulation. Use this one as a stepping-stone to other more arousing sexual positions, or to have fun with your lover by experimenting with different sensations.

Some couples may feel this is rather an impersonal method of lovemaking But if she turns her head and body slightly she too can see her posterior rising and falling. Alternatively, make love in front of a mirror so that you can both get the voyeuristic thrill of watching each other.

thigh cocoon

Treat your man to a sensory feast in this sexy position

The woman raises her legs and keeps her thighs pressed tightly together, creating a cocoon for his penis. During sex, the woman does most of the work, producing exquisite sensations for both partners.

The woman lies back and raises her feet up straight above the man's shoulders so that he can kneel in front of her to penetrate. Her calves and feet are within easy reach of his hands, so he can caress them or hold them to steady himself while thrusting vigorously from beneath. To build up her excitement he can use his fingers to caress her clitoris and perineum.

In this position the woman can grasp her partner's hips with her hands to pull him toward her. This increases the friction between the vagina and penis, and so heightens the intensity of her, and his, excitement.

This is a satisfying position for the man if he likes to watch his woman take control. And since she is controlling the action, she can make her movements as fast or slow as she chooses.

• DRAW OUT AROUSAL

Spend time pleasuring each others' bodies with your hands, lips, and tongues before going for orgasm. As a result of a long, sensitive build-up, your climaxes will be longer and stronger. The more excitement you create along the way, the greater the climax will be when it finally arrives.

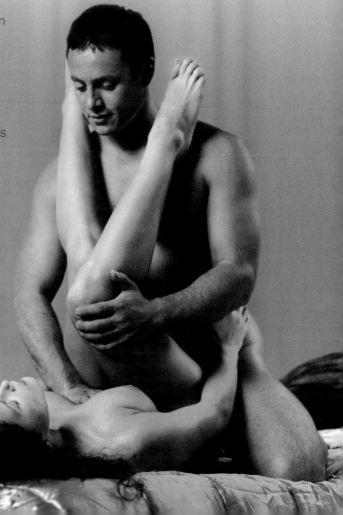

the cat

Make your woman purr in this submissive position

It is not surprising that rear-entry positions feature frequently in our fantasies. The buttocks generate strong sexual signals, which are heightened during lovemaking.

Here, the woman comfortably rests on her knees and elbows and parts her legs wide enough to allow her partner to kneel between them. He places his hands on the small of her back, penetrates, then draws her backward and forward on to his penis.

This is a naturally pleasurable position for him, and she can lower or raise her position to match his height by leaning up or down on her forearms and arching her back—like a cat. And at the same time, she can reach between her legs to stroke her clitoris.

In this position the man is stable enough for him to have his hands free, so that he can caress her buttocks, back, and breasts. Consequently, this is one of the most satisfying of all the rear-entry positions.

• SENSUAL BATHING

Take a sensual bath with your lover. Settle into the warm water and use a sudsy gel to wash each other slowly and sensuously. Let your fingers slip into each other's most secret places, and use your slippery hands and fingers to arouse sensations all over each other's skin, leaving you both perfectly prepared for sex.

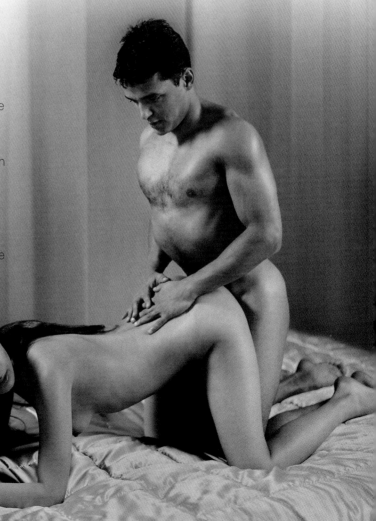

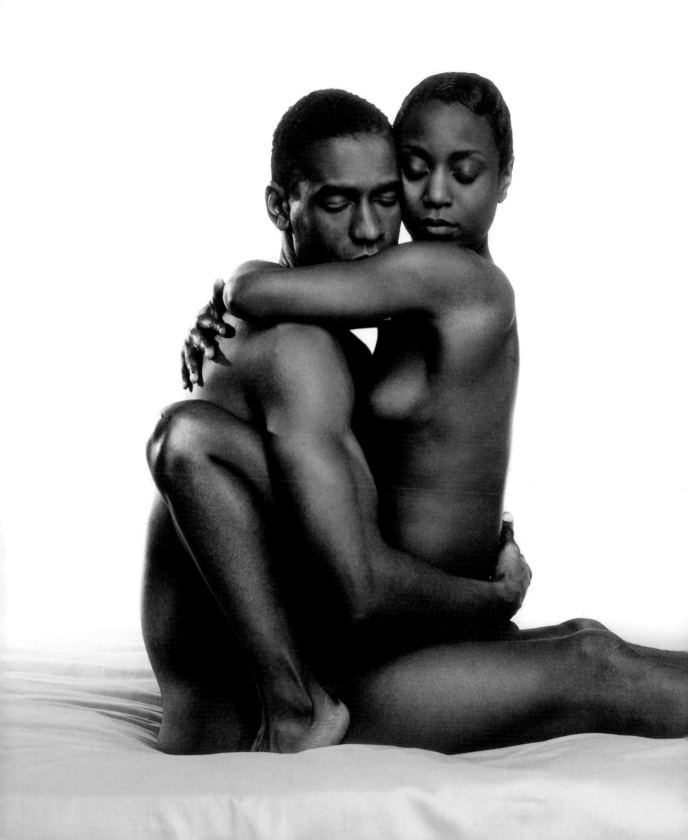

woman in repose

Get face-to-face in this sexy position designed for her pleasure

Any face-to-face position feels supremely intimate and erotic, especially when you are squeezed up against your lover's body. This woman-on-top position gives both lovers great sensations.

The man remains fairly still and sits with his legs outstretched, while the woman sits astride him and guides his penis into her vagina. He wraps his arms around her and supports her body as she moves.

The woman sets the pace of lovemaking here—and power is, after all, an aphrodisiac. She can choose to sit in simple repose while you both concentrate on the sensations of physical closeness. Or she can use her feet to provide leverage for her thrusts, although she may not be able to maintain this for long. As the man surrenders to his partner's movements, his pleasure will increase every time she slides down on to his penis, particularly if she grips him with her muscles.

This position is also incredibly arousing for her, as his penis should stimulate her clitoris, plus any of her vaginal hot spots that she chooses. Combined with being tightly embraced and caressed by her lover, this position could result in a multiple orgasm.

Not all women experience multiple orgasms, but a lot more manage it than their male counterparts. Multiple climaxes consist of a series of separate orgasms—these might be small or large peaks—occurring within a short time. To experience a multiple orgasm, a woman must experience continued stimulation after her initial climax. Men: if necessary, move into another position after she has climaxed so you can keep stimulating her.

• SHARE SENSUAL EXPERIENCES

Even when you and your partner have learned to discover your options, there is still room for expanding your sexual knowledge of each other. Sharing sensual experiences is about keeping your sexual excitement for each other alive. Do this by trying a new sexual position every few weeks, or masturbating in front of your lover. When you have time, take a bath or shower together, then massage each other with scented oils and give a foot massage. Other sensual experiences you might like to try include brushing and washing each other's hair, eating dinner together in the nude, finger-painting each other's bodies, reading erotica together, or out loud to each other, and sharing a vibrator (see pages 164–165) for added sexual thrills.

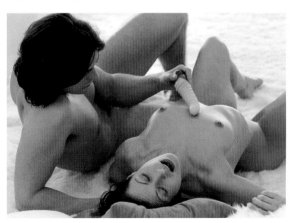

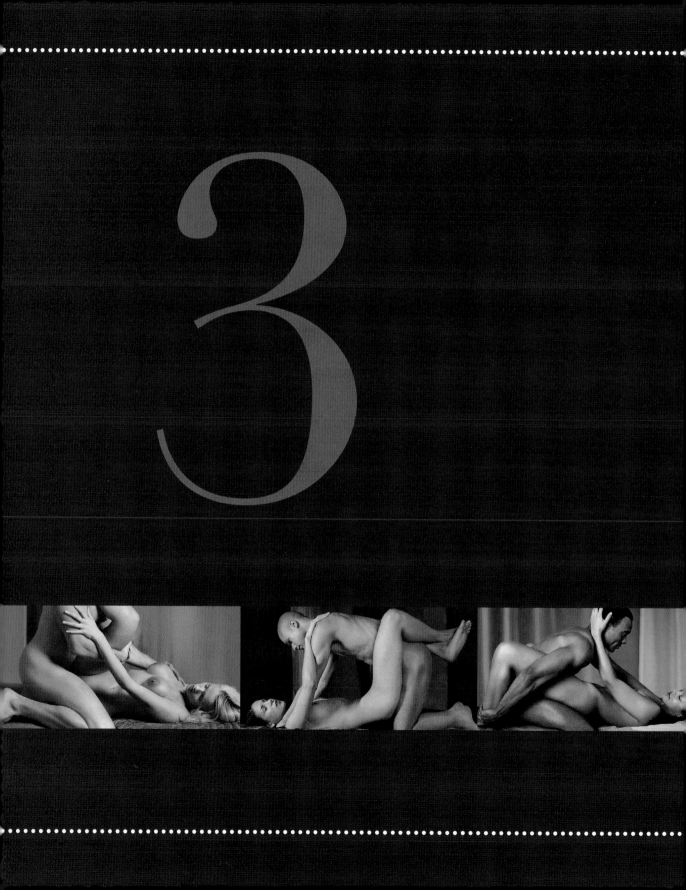

Acrobatic Ecstasy

Given the opportunity, many people would like secretly to watch another couple making love. Men in particular are interested in the shapes and poses of sex, perhaps because their acute visual senses respond so stirringly to what they see. These positions will encourage you to try new ways of sexually gratifying your lover, and by learning how to increase your sensations during sex, you can greatly intensify your own sexual experience.

These positions will challenge you and your partner to open up your minds and bodies. Stretch yourself in the Lotus-like position or Splitting Bamboo. Discover new angles of penetration in Gripping with Toes or Tail of the Ostrich. Lose yourself in arousing positions such as Bareback Rider, or create a sexual sculpture in Joined at the Hip.

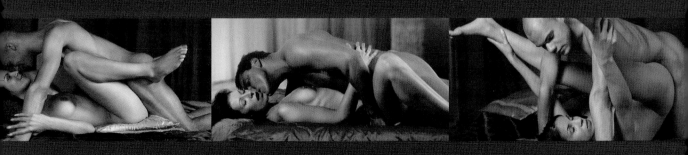

• STAYING FLEXIBLE

A common obstacle to good sex, particularly in later life, is joint inflexibility and stiffness, both of which mean that you can't move in the way you want to during lovemaking. Two great methods of staying toned, flexible, and mobile are yoga and Pilates. Both are gentle and safe forms of exercise that emphasize the importance of posture, core-strength, alignment, and breathing. Pilates is a relaxing and relatively easy way to strengthen and maintain core strength, and can help to tone vaginal floor muscles. Yoga is helpful because the poses form part of a meditation that can help to relax your body and focus your mind.

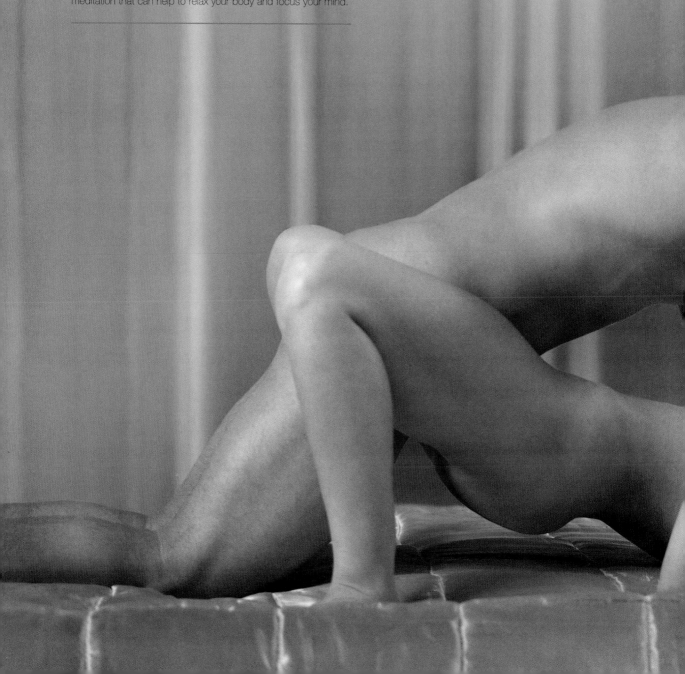

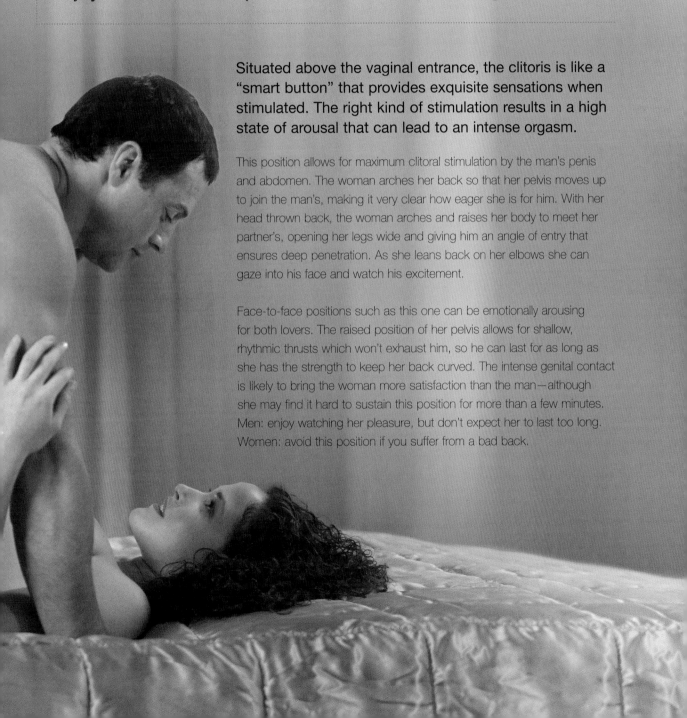

stimulating the clitoris

Enjoy intense clitoral pleasure in this back-bending position

Situated above the vaginal entrance, the clitoris is like a "smart button" that provides exquisite sensations when stimulated. The right kind of stimulation results in a high state of arousal that can lead to an intense orgasm.

This position allows for maximum clitoral stimulation by the man's penis and abdomen. The woman arches her back so that her pelvis moves up to join the man's, making it very clear how eager she is for him. With her head thrown back, the woman arches and raises her body to meet her partner's, opening her legs wide and giving him an angle of entry that ensures deep penetration. As she leans back on her elbows she can gaze into his face and watch his excitement.

Face-to-face positions such as this one can be emotionally arousing for both lovers. The raised position of her pelvis allows for shallow, rhythmic thrusts which won't exhaust him, so he can last for as long as she has the strength to keep her back curved. The intense genital contact is likely to bring the woman more satisfaction than the man—although she may find it hard to sustain this position for more than a few minutes. Men: enjoy watching her pleasure, but don't expect her to last too long. Women: avoid this position if you suffer from a bad back.

lotus-like

Challenge your sexual boundaries with this yoga-style position

The sheer eroticism of this position will probably be a turn-on for him. The tangle of limbs writhing beneath him, and the openess of his lover's vagina, are likely to make him submit to her, body and soul.

The woman crosses her legs and tucks each foot under the opposite knee in the lotus position, then draws her feet up to rest on her torso. The man leans over to penetrate her in this position. In theory, the result of adopting this familiar yoga pose is to draw

the vagina up to meet the penis. During sex, her legs form a barrier to prevent him penetrating her very deeply. His shallow strokes reign in his excitement, and can graze her clitoris to add to her pleasure, giving both partners a long, slow burn to orgasm.

This position is designed for supple women with some experience of yoga, and most who try it find they can't hold it for long. Nevertheless, the excitement of it might convince you to get in training just for the thrill of trying it out on your man.

• THRUSTING MOTIONS

Men: don't restrict yourself to in-out lovemaking motions. Use your penis to sensually awaken your lover by rubbing it along one side of her vagina, or pushing forcefully against it. Change tempo and move your penis rapidly and lightly in and out of her, penetrating the vagina from above, and pushing against her clitoris.

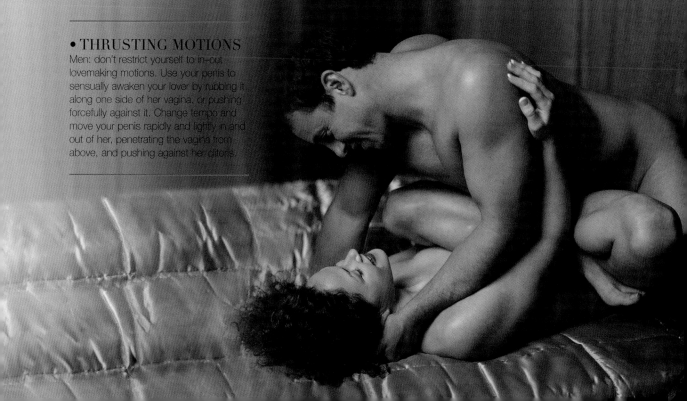

leg stretch

Stretch out and enjoy super sensations in this ballet-like pose

This position looks more like a movement in a gymnastics display than hot, whole-hearted passion. But it is easier than it looks, and the deep penetration he achieves can be arousing for both lovers.

Stretching itself is a sexy activity, and couples might move naturally into this position after trying the "thigh cocoon" (see page 96). Here, the woman lifts one of her feet and stretches her leg out past her partner's body. She bends the other leg at the knee, placing the sole of her foot on his chest.

Most women find the action of stretching their legs during sex to be intensely erotic. This position also exposes her clitoris, to allow her more stimulation. She can further intensify her arousal by rolling her pelvis up against her man's.

Women: this position constricts the vagina which feels great, but ask your lover to avoid thrusting too hard or you may feel more discomfort than pleasure.

• HARMONIOUS SOUNDS

Soft, soothing music, such as flute music, harmonious new-age sounds, and many of Mozart's inimitable pieces, infiltrate the many layers of human consciousness and evoke a relaxed, open, and receptive mood—perfect for sensual lovemaking.

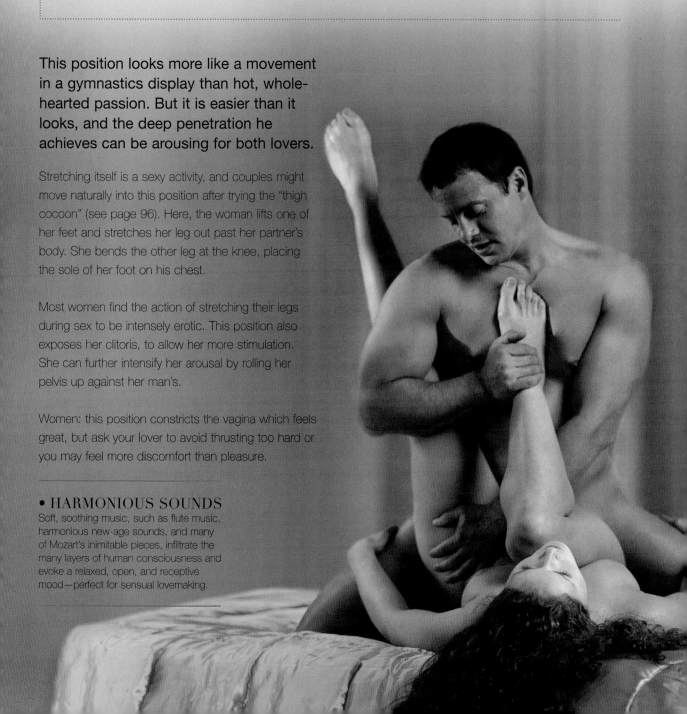

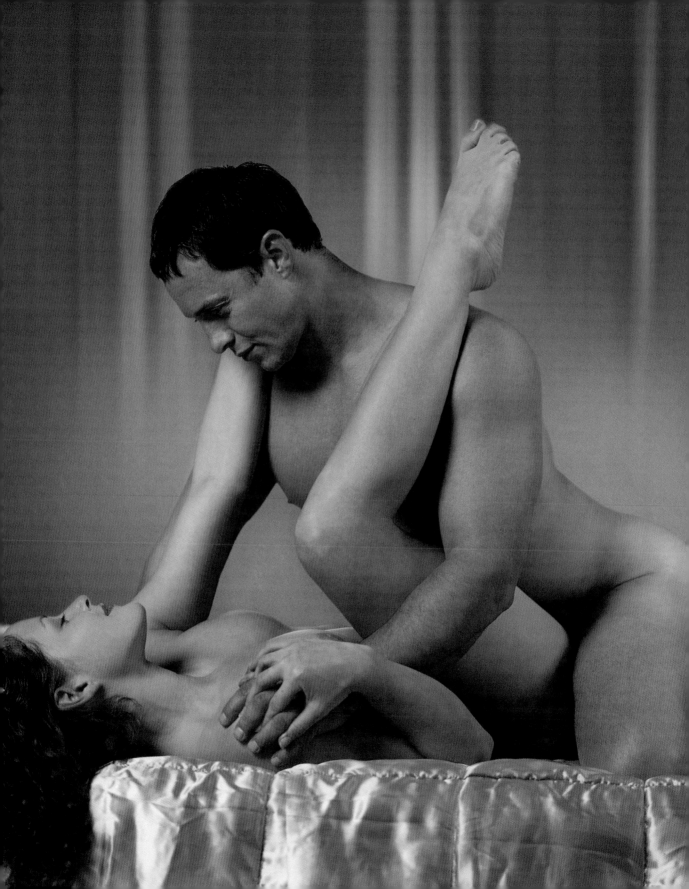

erotic fold

Energize your sex life with this fun—if acrobatic—position

Erotic positions such as this one are reminiscent of a new couple in the first intense moments of their relationship, inventing and reinventing crazy new lovemaking positions.

By trying out new positions and new techniques, lovers can discover thrilling new sensations, and that's a surefire way of spicing up your usual lovemaking routines. By being adventurous, long-term or older couples can rediscover a little young-love excitement to refresh their relationship.

In this acrobatic position, the woman lies back and lifts her legs to rest over her man's shoulders while he penetrates her from a kneeling position. During lovemaking, she raises one leg and puts it on her partner's shoulder, then brings that leg down and raises the other. The sequence is repeated again and again, requiring considerable suppleness.

As the woman raises each leg in turn, her lover's penis is squeezed first by one set of vaginal muscles, then another, producing intense sensations. As her vagina tightens and releases, the action of clenching her vaginal muscles builds up pressure in her pelvis.

This lovemaking position will enable both lovers to enjoy a long, drawn-out arousal. He can slow down his orgasm and give her pleasure by stopping

intermittently to stroke her clitoris or caress and kiss her foot or ankle. Many women and men find foot touching intimate and sexually arousing, and she can also benefit from the changing angles of penetration. The main reward of this position for the woman is the knowledge that it makes her man feel wonderful.

• ENHANCED AROUSAL

Everyone knows that sex is enhanced by a long, sensual build-up. If couples want to arouse each other fully they can use the following guide to ensure their lovemaking has a slow, subtle prelude, to help improve both lovers' orgasms. Start by stroking and touching each other. After arousing yourselves, give closer physical contact in the form of playful rolling around and cuddling to heighten your desire. While cuddling, extend your loveplay to include mutual masturbation, but resist the temptation to have sex too soon. The last phase in your build up to sex could be giving each other an erotic tongue bath (see page 84) followed by oral sex. This will bring you both to a peak of physical longing, and set the scene for sensational orgasms.

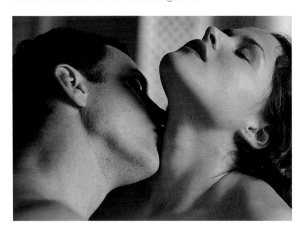

gripping with toes

Discover new angles of penetration and extend your lovemaking

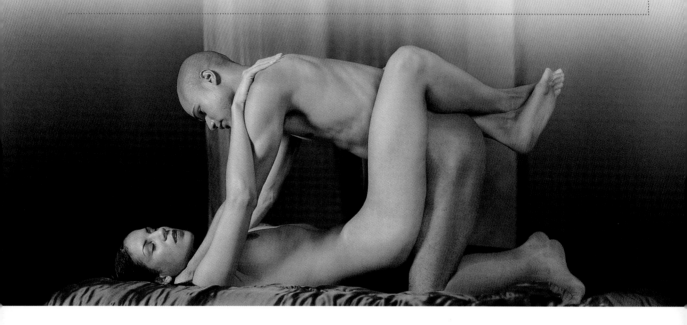

Changing position or altering the angle of penetration slows down lovemaking, and this can help to produce more intense orgasms for both of you.

This position is best used as a transition pose from one move to another, or as an interlude between more vigorous lovemaking. Its gentler pace allows you to focus on the intensity of your sensations.

The woman lies on her back while her man kneels between her thighs, places his hands either side of her neck, and braces himself with his toes to keep his balance. She wraps her legs tightly around his waist to pull herself up onto his penis.

Although the man is unable to thrust freely in this position, he can vary the angle of penetration by leaning toward or away from his woman. His long, slow thrusts can intensely stimulate her clitoris, while her leg-clinging embrace is erotic for both partners.

• SQUEEZE TECHNIQUE
Women: if your man reaches "the point of no return" but wants to prolong lovemaking, he can prevent himself from climaxing by squeezing his penis hard on the coronal ridge between his fingers and thumb. You can also use this technique on him. When your man tells you that he's reaching bursting point, apply the squeeze, then massage his erection back to life by stroking his genitals or using your mouth. This means that you can continue enjoying sex until he is ready to climax again.

---

ankle hold

Flex your legs wide and roll up to seduce your man

This athletic pose looks more like a workout than a lovemaking position, but it is recommended for the man who has a short penis—and a flexible lover.

The woman lies on her back and raises her legs. She draws her legs back and holds them apart with her hands, allowing her man to lean over her and move in close. He kneels by her hips and places his hands on either side of her head for support before entering her.

If the man has a short penis, he will find that he gains extra stimulation from penetrating his partner's vagina when it is constricted in this position.

For most women, however, this is a supremely uncomfortable position to sustain. Let him know when you want to move into more mutually satisfying lovemaking. To get more stimulation from one-sided positions like this, couples can investigate alternatives such as mutual masturbation, oral sex, or sex aids.

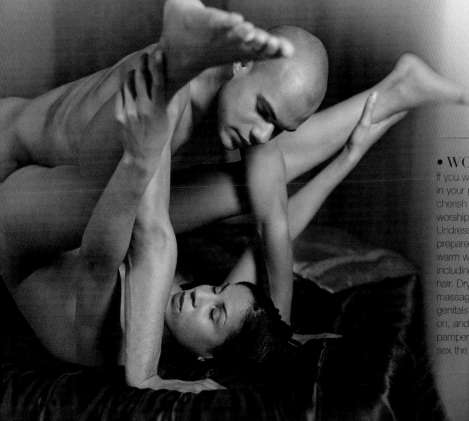

• WORSHIP YOUR MAN

If you want to generate fantastic feelings in your partner, and encourage him to cherish you in return, here's a male worship ritual that you both might enjoy. Undress your partner, lead him to a prepared bath, and settle him into the warm water. Carefully wash his body, including his genitals, and shampoo his hair. Dry him with warm towels, then massage his body with oil. Caress his genitals. Tell him how much he turns you on, and how you love his body. End the pampering session by giving him oral or sex the way he likes it best.

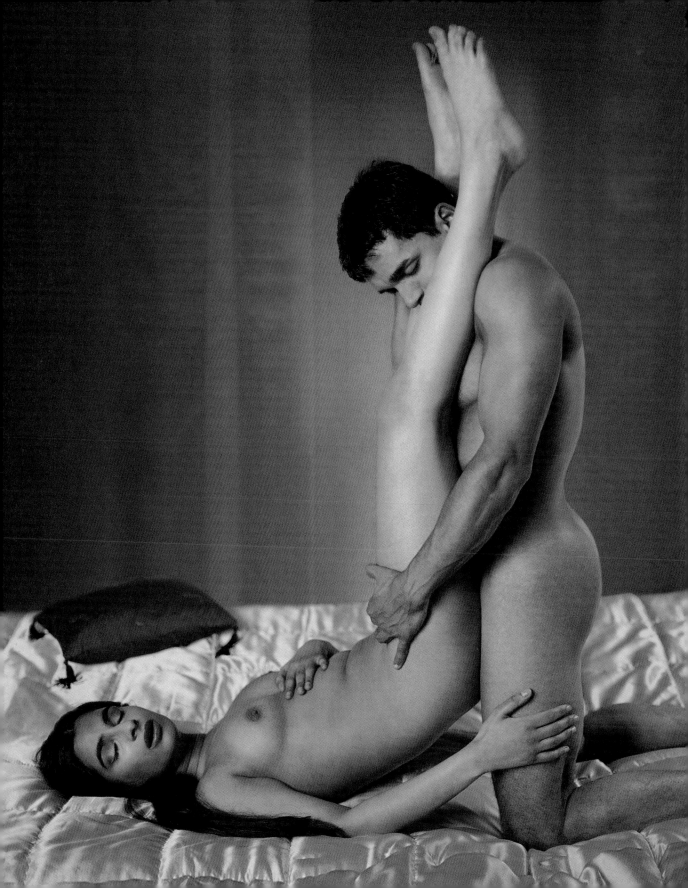

tail of the ostrich

Raise your legs and indulge your man with this erotic treat

Other lovemaking positions might offer couples more pleasure than this one, but the eroticism of achieving this unusual posture is a reward in itself.

The woman lies back on the bed with her legs raised, while her man kneels up behind her hips. He lifts her legs and holds them to his chest as he enters her.

To intensify her pleasure, the man can squeeze her buttocks together with his thighs so that her vagina is pressed firmly around his penis. He can vary her sensations by raising or lowering her hips to alter the depth and angle of penetration. As he does this, he should support the small of her back with his hand.

For the woman, the most benefit to be gained from this position is probably the rush of blood to her head from being upside down, which can actually intensify excitement and orgasm. This posture doesn't provide much clitoral stimulation, so try moving into it after a particularly stimulating position or immediately following oral sex.

Couples might like to combine this position with the "lover's grip" (see page 23), in which the woman's buttocks rest on the man's lap and her legs lie over his shoulders. After penetrating in that position, which is intensely pleasurable for both partners, the couple can move into this more advanced pose to slow down sex and delay climax. Use the variation to concentrate on small but sublime differences in stimulation. By varying the angle of penetration, these positions, which can be performed as a sequence during lovemaking, give both partners a variety of deeply pleasurable sensations.

• DEER EXERCISE FOR WOMEN

The Deer Exercise originated in ancient China, and is thought to strengthen the female system, balance hormones, stave off signs of aging, and energize the glands, bringing harmony and health throughout the body. It consists of two sets of exercises to be carried out daily. In the first stage, sit with the heel of your foot pressed up against your vagina to give a firm pressure on the clitoris. Next, rub your hands together vigorously to make them hot. Stroke your breasts in slow circular motions outward for a minimum of 36 times, and a maximum of 360 times, twice a day. In the second stage, which can be done either sitting or lying down, flex your vaginal muscles in a similar fashion to Kegel exercises (see page 87). At the same time, massage your labia.

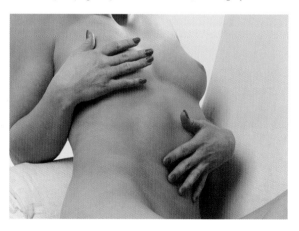

leg crossover

Intensify his sensations by crossing your leg over his chest

This position requires a certain amount of suppleness, but introduces an element of sexual exploration into your lovemaking, which couples may find mutually exciting.

The woman lies on her side, although the pose is marginally less difficult if she lies on her back. The man sits back on his heels with one of her legs over his shoulder and the other between his thighs. He gently thrusts from a kneeling position while the woman uses her vaginal muscles to stimulate his penis.

A supple woman can enhance both lovers' sensations by moving her leg from one shoulder to the other in sequence. This action opens and closes her vagina around his penis, allowing for deeper penetration. Using her hands or a fingertip vibrator to stimulate her clitoris can greatly enhance her pleasure in this position, and so intensify climax for both partners.

• FANTASY FETISHES
One of the major sexual differences between men and women is that men are more prone to develop fetishes—about shoes or breasts, for example. This doesn't mean he is compelled to act on them in reality, but they can form an active part of his sexual imagination, particularly in positions like this one.

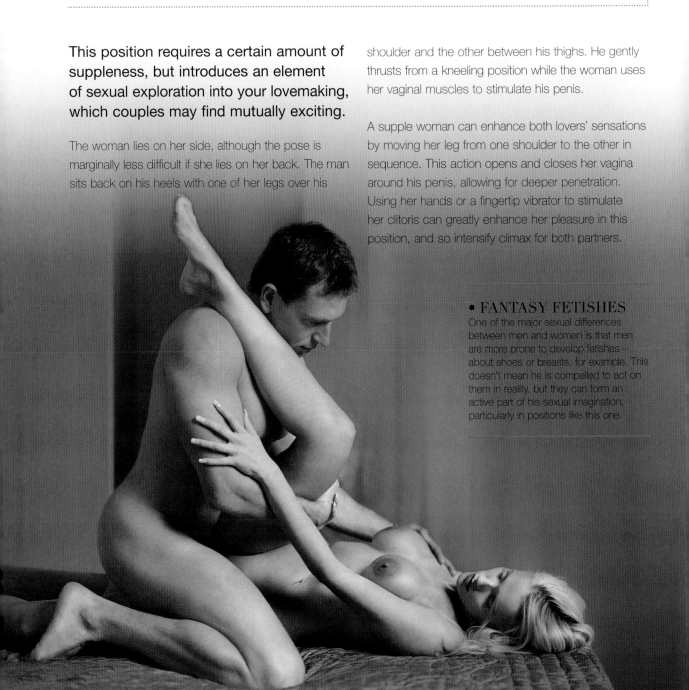

divinely deep

Enjoy deeply satisfying sex in this arousing lovemaking position

This erotic pose looks acrobatic, but is easy to attain and comfortable. The depth of penetration means intense stimulation for both partners, but she'll need to be fully aroused to enjoy sex in this position.

The woman lies on her back and lifts her knees to her chest, placing her calves on his shoulders. Her man kneels close to her and supports himself on his arms to penetrate her deeply.

If she pulls her knees up and back, the woman can greatly increase the depth of his penetration, but he'll need to thrust very gently to avoid hurting her.

She may increase her pleasure by holding onto his buttocks and moving her pelvis up to meet his. This rocking action can stimulate her clitoris, and allow deep vaginal pressure. The rhythmic sensations stimulate the length of his penis and make him feel entirely enclosed inside her—very sensual indeed.

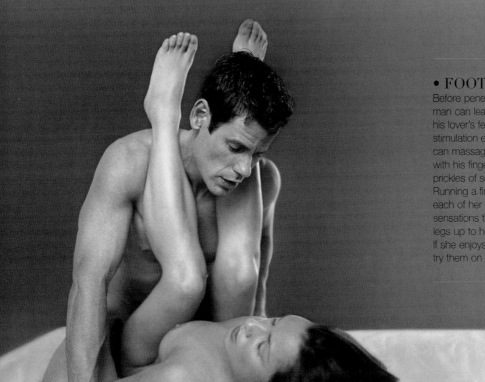

• FOOT MASSAGE

Before penetrating in this position, the man can lean back on his heels and rub his lover's feet. Many women find foot stimulation extremely erotic. To start, he can massage the area under her toes with his fingers to provoke powerful prickles of sensuality throughout her body. Running a finger sensuously between each of her toes can transmit erotic sensations through nerves all along her legs up to her inner thighs and genitals. If she enjoys these sensations, she might try them on him to test his response.

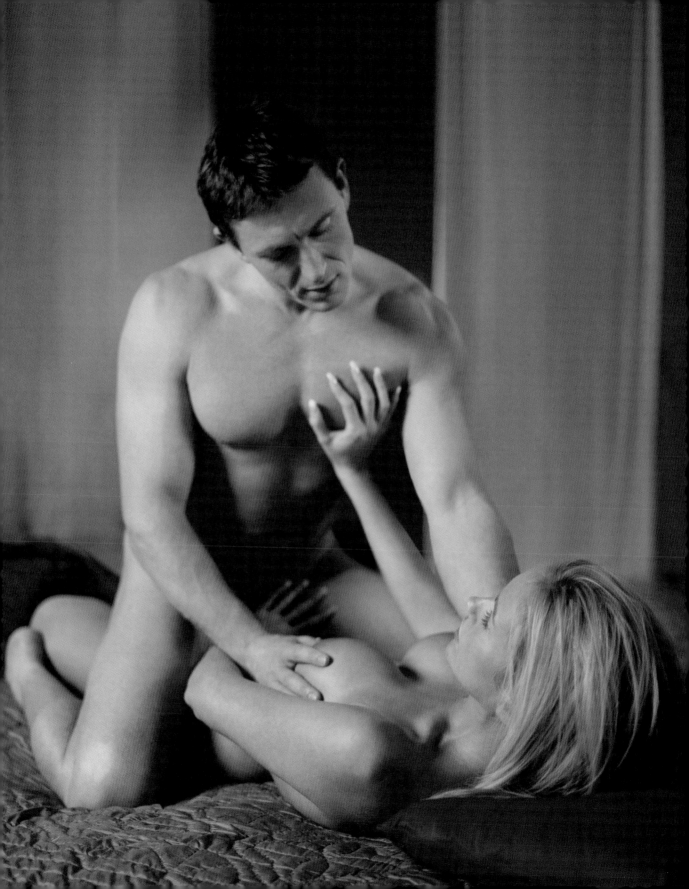

yoga poser

Electrify your man's senses with this sexy, yoga-style position

Women may enjoy great sensations in this position, but will need to be very supple to perform it. The rewards of this posture may even inspire you to take up yoga.

This position has two variations. She can either lie with her thighs open and her ankles crossed, as though performing the lotus position, while her man kneels astride her; or she can cross her legs and pull them back before he enters her, so that her legs rest against his chest (see page 104). Both positions ensure maximum clitoral stimulation and deep penetration.

Each of the variations of this cross-legged posture has its own benefits. Pulling her legs back allows for deep penetration and G-spot stimulation, while crossing her ankles can improve clitoral stimulation. In either case, her lover's hands are free to caress her body, and she can use her fingertips to scratch and stroke his chest.

This face-to-face position is also very stimulating and comfortable for the man. He can use his hands to support her back, or stroke her neck and breasts. If the man wants to heighten his pleasure, he should ask his woman to change the position of her hips to enable him to vary the angle and depth of penetration.

A certain level of fitness is required, however, for the woman to get into position, but there are many obvious health benefits to staying fit and trim. Sexual responses can also benefit from improved fitness. Toned abdominal muscles, improved core-strength, and stronger thighs can allow more intense sexual arousal, heightened response, and deeper orgasms in both men and women. In addition, regularly practicing Kegel exercises (see page 87) will help to strengthen a woman's vaginal muscles, which means they will contract more dramatically during orgasm. This can heighten sexual pleasure for both partners.

• NIPPLE PLAY FOR HIM

Women: while you are in this position, use your hands in a swimming motion—as if doing breast stroke—over your man's chest. Then run your fingers softly around his nipples, and brush your fingertips from side to side across the top, so that your fingers actually leave the nipples before going back in the opposite direction. He may be excited by the way his body reacts to these delicate sensations, even more so if you begin these actions slowly, then speed up.

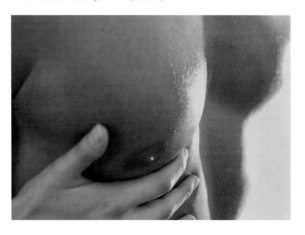

tantric sex

This spiritual approach to sex aims to enrich the mind and soul as well as provide extreme sensual pleasure. Although Tantric touch may feel the same as other forms of touch, there is a different emphasis on how it is given and received. Tantra emphasizes "touch for pleasure's sake," stressing the importance of giving and receiving pleasure in a certain way. A priority of Tantric sex is to prolong sexual arousal by extensive stroking sessions followed by very slow intercourse.

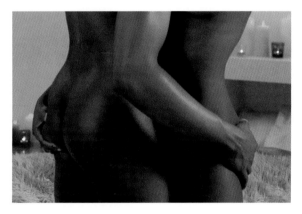

Stand facing each other, stare into each other's eyes, and try not to speak. Begin by slowly stroking your partner's neck, shoulders, back, buttocks, and legs.

Touch each other's genitals very lightly—this stroking is not meant to result in orgasm. Remember to stroke his testicles and perineum, and her vagina, labia, and clitoris.

Tantric strokes

Start by lightly stroking each other, first with a circling action, then up and down. Avoid the breasts and the genitals at this stage.

Stroke slowly for about 15 minutes, take a break, then repeat for another 15 minutes. Later, repeat the stroking for 30 minutes. Lie quietly together in the spoons position, but without stimulating each other (if this is too tempting, lie facing each other with foreheads together, but bodies not quite touching).

Intimate stroking

Next, make light, circular movements on the chest or breast, first with hands moving toward each other, then with the action reversed.

Move on to the genitals, slowly drawing your hands or fingers up from underneath them using light strokes, and working along the length of the penis or up the height of the vulva. After an hour of genital stroking, take a five-minute break. Then lie motionless, with the woman on top and the man's penis inside her vagina, until his erection subsides.

Tantric intercourse

Only once you've completed the Tantric strokes do you move on to intercourse—the key is to take your time (orgasm should be put off for at least 20 minutes to half an hour).

The penis should penetrate the vagina by only a few inches or so, stay there for a full minute, then withdraw and rest in the clitoral hood for a further minute before sliding back in. Each penetration should be followed by a full minute's rest. For the next few strokes, let the penis rest outside the vulva, then on subsequent strokes just inside it.

There are two sensations to be appreciated during Tantric lovemaking. The first is your own—what you feel when you touch your partner. The second is to imagine what your partner feels when touched by you.

There are various positions that are suitable for Tantric intercourse because they either prolong lovemaking or increase the pleasure of orgasm. To extend intercourse use a side-by-side or missionary position in which the man can control his impending orgasm by pulling his testicles downward. Alternatively, a woman-on-top position will increase her pleasure.

Rear-entry positions are also excellent for enhancing orgasm. The man can easily reach the woman's clitoris to stimulate her, and when she climaxes, his proximity to her anal muscles means that his penis will be affected by the strength of her contractions.

Woman-on-top positions are perfect for the slow, flowing movements of Tantric intercourse, and allow her to savor the sensations fully without distraction.

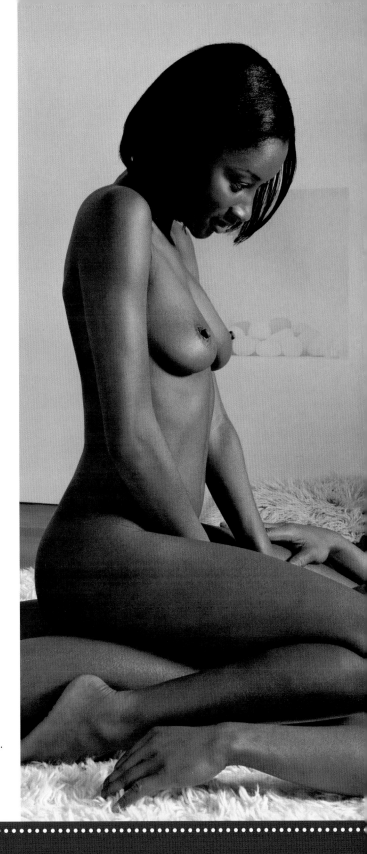

bareback rider

Extend your physical boundaries with this challenging position

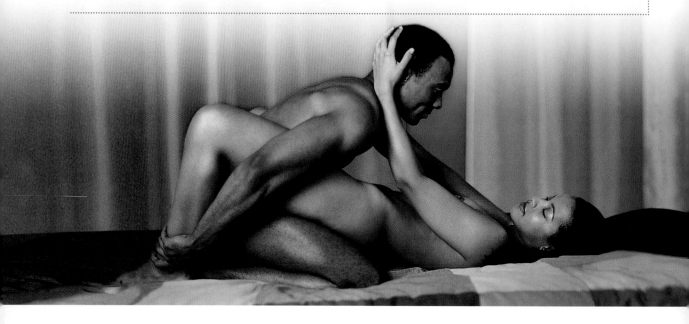

The man may find this position intensely exciting because it requires him to hold on to his woman's neck and foot like a rider clinging to a speeding horse.

The man kneels between his lover's legs with his thighs beneath her buttocks. She bends her knees to grasp him with her thighs, and tucks her feet in close to his. When he has entered her, he holds the back of her neck gently with one hand, pulls her foot or ankle close to him with the other hand, and begins to thrust.

The optimum way to make love in this complicated posture is to move up and down, but this could prove difficult if the man is tall and the woman is small and

light. The upside is that this position feels very athletic and exciting for both partners, and the man may enjoy controlling or riding his woman. Provided she is happy to submit to him, the woman can enjoy the sensation of having her limbs stretched during lovemaking. Women: if you can relax into this one, you'll enjoy deep penetration, and vigorous stimulation.

• CIRCLING EXERCISE
This a great exercise for women and men to improve hip and pelvic mobility. Stand with your feet hip-width apart, and move your hips slowly in small circles. Gradually make the circles bigger and bigger, as if twirling a hula-hoop around your waist. Aim to make the circles as fluid and rhythmic as possible. A sexy variation of this exercise is to stand close to your partner, wrap your arms around each other, and rotate your hips in unison.

playful pleasure

Lose yourself in each other and in playful sensuality

This imaginative and playful position offers the possibility of deep penetration. As with all such positions, the man should spend time arousing his woman before penetrating, to ensure her pleasure.

The woman lies on her back and holds onto her ankles to expose her vagina. The woman is very accessible in this pose, and he can arouse her by using his penis to rub up and down her inner labia, then across or around her clitoris. Once she is fully aroused, he can penetrate her deeply from his kneeling position, maintaining intimacy by stroking the backs of her knees and thighs as he thrusts.

Both partners will enjoy the sexual friction created by this position, and may find that they reach climax easily, particularly if he uses his hands to stimulate her in rhythm with his deep thrusts.

Men: if your woman finds this lovemaking pose tiring, combine it with a more relaxing and intimate position, such as "flower in a vase" (see pages 60–61).

• DEER EXERCISE FOR MEN

This ancient Chinese exercise is believed to rejuvenate men by building up sexual tissue, increasing blood flow to the abdomen, drawing energy into the body, and balancing the sexual system. Stage one is to rub your palms together to generate warmth. Then, with your right hand, cup your testicles and place the palm of your left hand on your pubis. With a slight pressure move your left hand 81 times, then rub your hands together, and reverse the position using your right hand. Stage two is to contract and release your rectal muscles regularly, morning and evening.

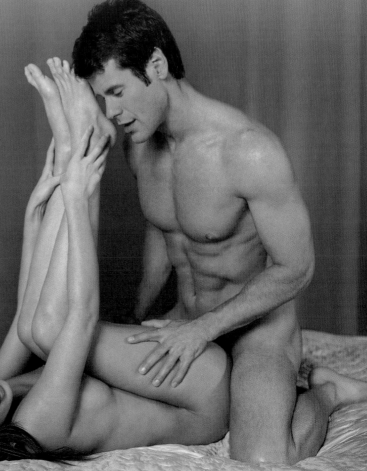

tightly enclosed

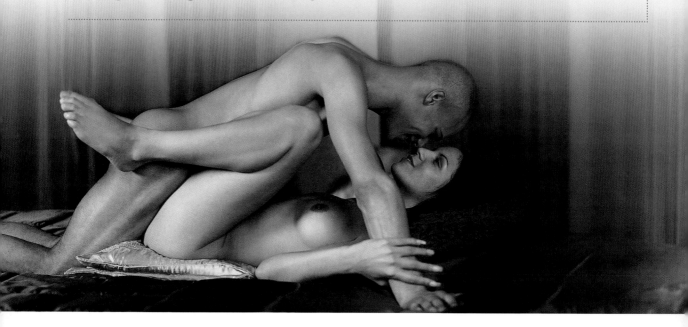

In this position, a woman can offer her man intense stimulation, and enjoy a sensation of fullness herself. Use this one when you're highly aroused and ready to experience deep vaginal stimulation.

The woman lies back and raises her knees, embracing his buttocks with her ankles. A cushion under her hips will help to support her back as she lies in this constricted position. The man kneels between her thighs and leans forward against her bent legs, pressing her knees toward her breasts. This action pushes the cervix forward, making penetration quite difficult, and thrusting his penis deep inside her.

The walls of her vagina will be pressed tightly together, gripping his penis so that he experiences very intense stimulation. She will feel a corresponding intensity of sensation—so much so that this position might be painful. If this is the case, it's time to move into a more mutually enjoyable position.

• THE FRENULUM

The penis has lots of ultra-sensitive spots, but stimulating his frenulum—the band-like ligament that links the ridge on the underside with the shaft—is particularly arousing. It's full of nerve endings, and just titillating the frenulum with your hand or tongue can make some men super-responsive. Make a ring with your hand around the ridge of his penis and move up and down using light, quick strokes. He should respond to this well.

---

joined at the hip

Create a sexual sculpture as you join in this erotic pose

The aim of pleasuring your lover is simply that—to give pleasure, not specifically to give orgasm. At times, the sensuality you generate can be so wonderful that orgasm may actually seem an anti-climax.

In this position, the woman lies on her left side and bends her right leg at the knee, pulling it up to hip-level with her hand. The man kneels behind his woman's hips, supporting her shoulder, and holds her leg up and across him to penetrate her.

The deep penetration and sexual friction the man achieves in this position will heighten his excitement and pleasure. When the woman pulls her leg right back, she stretches the vaginal area, which can make her feel exposed, vulnerable, and sensuous. This may be an erotic turn-on for both lovers.

Men: while thrusting, lightly massage underneath her shoulder blade using your fingertips. Many women have an extremely sensitive spot in this area, and stroking can enhance her erotic sensations.

• PENIS EXERCISE
Penis fitness can help a man to delay his orgasms and improve sexual responses. It can even help him achieve multiple orgasms. One pelvic-floor strengthening exercise is to "twitch" the penis 10 times a session for at least three sessions a day.

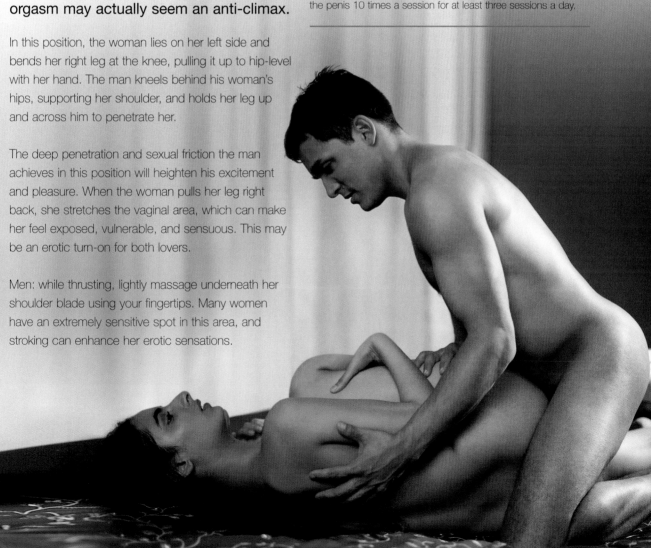

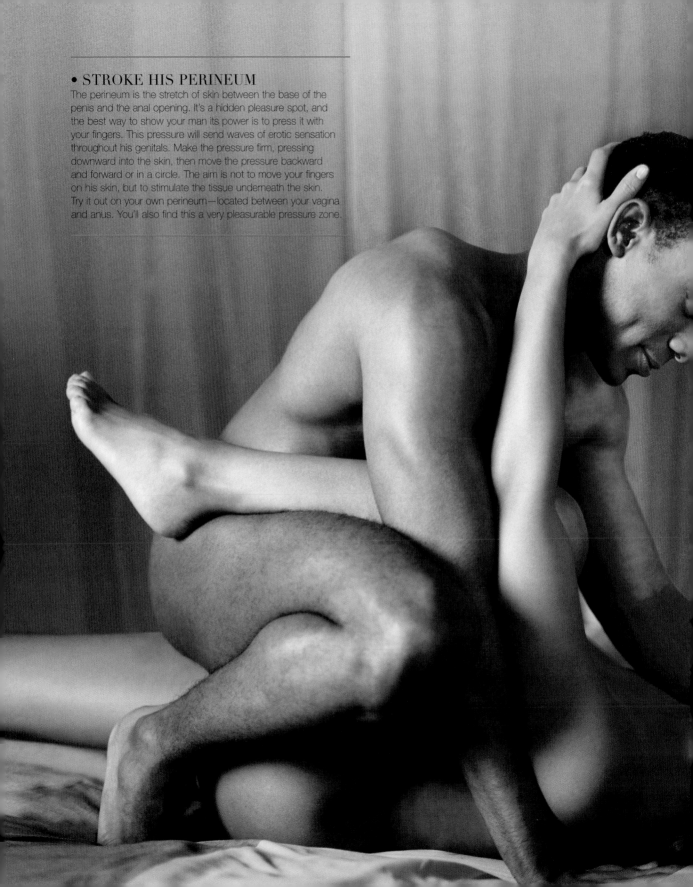

• STROKE HIS PERINEUM

The perineum is the stretch of skin between the base of the penis and the anal opening. It's a hidden pleasure spot, and the best way to show your man its power is to press it with your fingers. This pressure will send waves of erotic sensation throughout his genitals. Make the pressure firm, pressing downward into the skin, then move the pressure backward and forward or in a circle. The aim is not to move your fingers on his skin, but to stimulate the tissue underneath the skin. Try it out on your own perineum—located between your vagina and anus. You'll also find this a very pleasurable pressure zone.

kneeling squat

Thrill your lover by standing over her in this athletic pose

There are many fabulous ways to enjoy a great time in bed, and the more we learn about human sexual response the more we understand the desirability of experimenting with every method of good loving.

Here, the woman lies on her back with her right leg stretched out. Leaning over slightly to the right, she bends her left knee and raises her leg. The man faces her and sits on top of her thighs. He rests his weight on his left leg by kneeling on the bed or squatting (although he'll need strong legs). He then bends his right knee, and moves his right leg forward under his lover's raised left leg and penetrates her from this position. His weight rests slightly on her thighs, and there is something bird-like and friendly about his squat.

Her raised leg exposes her clitoris to friction as he thrusts, which she may find intensely pleasurable. Both lovers may find themselves tuning into and heightening each others' passion in this creative position. He may find it difficult to maintain his balance for very long, but this makes the perfect interlude from more conventional lovemaking positions.

By being imaginative and changing your lovemaking scenario from time to time, you can extend your emotional and physical knowledge of each other. Always try experimenting with different positions, both in bed and elsewhere, and break away from the idea that sex should only be done at night by making love at other times.

sensational shake

Get ready to play with your lover in this friendly position

This is a good position for older men who may tire quickly in strenuous man-on-top positions. It creates good sensations for both partners, but it does require a little flexibility in the female partner.

The woman lies on her back and places one foot up over her partner's shoulder. She draws back the other leg close to her body, so that her knee is by her shoulder. As long as her legs are flexible, this is a restful position for both partners, and the openness of the woman's body ensures plenty of sexual friction. Her foot can rest on her man's chest while he moves.

The man kneels upright to penetrate her, and is able to thrust deeply in this position. The angle and the depth of penetration will serve to increase the erotic tension. She also has one hand free to caress his body, to heighten her man's senses during lovemaking.

If the woman shakes the foot of her bent leg from time to time during penetration, it can add an extra frisson to the lovemaking, but she must be careful not to knock her man over—or even out.

• PELVIC-FLOOR FOR HIM

Most women know about the advantages of regularly practicing Kegel exercises, but men can also reap the sexual benefits of a tightly toned pelvic floor. Strong muscles will assist them achieve and maintain a firm erection. Some men also find that drawing up the pelvic-floor muscles can stop the urge to ejaculate, helping them to last longer during sex. Men: exercise your Kegel muscles by tensing them as hard as you can, and work up to holding this contraction for 10 seconds. Then let go and relax. Repeat this squeezing action up to 12 times, concentrating on holding the contraction at its height. Do this exercise several times a day, but stop if it becomes painful.

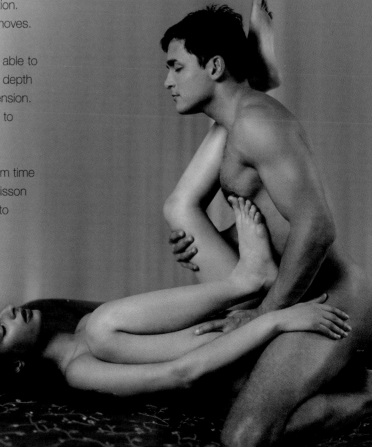

love's desire

This pose is definitely one to try for a man who has a fetish for legs or feet, but the erotic sensation of stretching and being stretched can also feel good for her.

By placing her heel on her partner's forehead, the woman's stretched leg stretches her vagina and perineum. As he thrusts, her raised leg will move in time, varying the degree of tension between vagina and penis and providing a range of sensations.

Watching each other in this pose feels exciting, and he can increase her pleasure—and his—by stroking her thighs and breasts. This position may be more satisfying for her if she strokes her clitoris as he thrusts.

After a while, her stretched leg may tire, and not every man is mad about having a foot resting against his forehead. When it's time for a change of position, she can move her leg down to rest over his thigh without interrupting lovemaking.

• MUTUAL SEXUAL DISCOVERY

This is a six-point plan to extend your mutual sexual knowledge. Lie side-by-side in bed and caress each other without touching genitals. Give each other a body massage (see pages 42–43). Stimulate each others' erogenous zones by kissing, licking, biting, and massaging them. Give body stimulus to his penis: try rubbing it between her breasts, thighs, or against her pubis. Give body stimulus to the vagina: try thrusting against his thigh, face, or buttocks. Finally, try having sex without climaxing, which means avoiding those positions known to lead rapidly to orgasm.

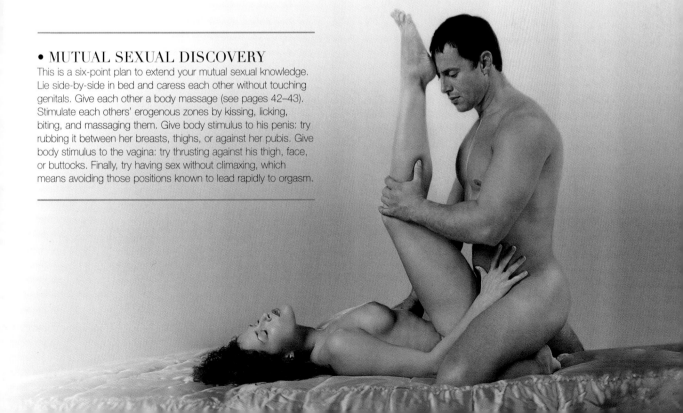

• EROGENOUS ZONES

The erogenous zones are the parts of the human body that feel particularly sensual when stroked, licked, kissed, or lightly bitten. Every person's hot spots are different—what feels sensual to one may feel ticklish to another or lack sensation to a third. The most sensitive areas are usually the mouth, ears, breasts, abdomen, insides of the thighs, genitals, feet, and toes, but we all vary widely, so it's a good idea to explore your partner's body in order to know what turns him, or her, on.

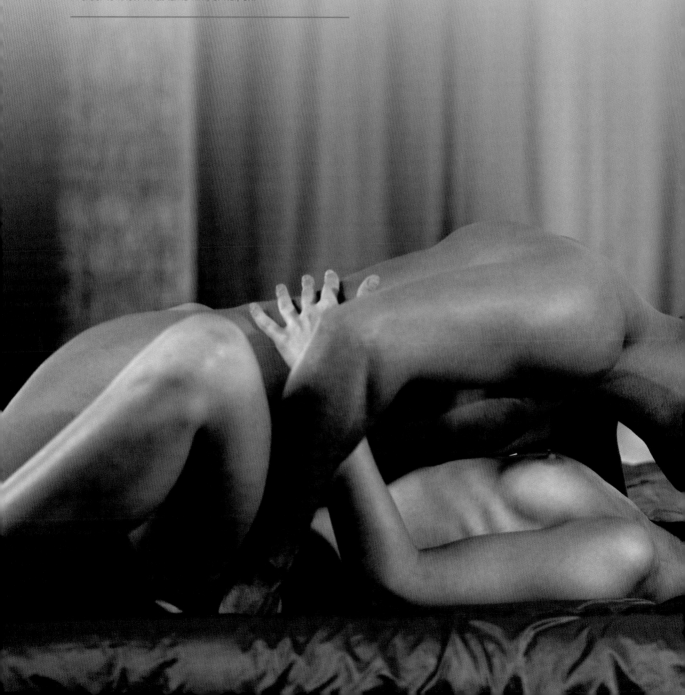

turning position

There's no law to say you should remain stuck in one position during lovemaking. Many couples vary their movements spontaneously. Here, the couple begins in the missionary position, but the man then makes a 180-degree turn without withdrawing his penis.

Understandably, this position takes a little practice. Even when perfected, it may not create the most erotic sensations, but couples can certainly feel that they have pushed the boundaries of sensuality.

Throughout the sequence, the man supports himself on his arms to hold his torso clear of his partner. Beginning in the missionary position, with his legs between the woman's, and without withdrawing his penis, the man lifts his right, then left leg over the woman's left leg. The woman can help by supporting his chest with her hands.

The man moves his legs until his body is at a right angle to his partner's. She should part her legs slightly to make it easier for him to remain inside her. The man continues to turn his torso around until he is facing her feet with his legs on either side of her body.

As the man turns, so the angle of his penetration changes, creating a range of different sensations on her clitoris and G-spot. She can reward him for his efforts by stroking his body as he turns, so that he enjoys an all-over body massage as he penetrates.

This position will appeal to anyone who enjoys sexual exploration, and it can lighten the mood of lovemaking. No one decreed that sex has to be serious. Have fun with this one, and enjoy the different sensation it creates between you—even if it is mostly laughter.

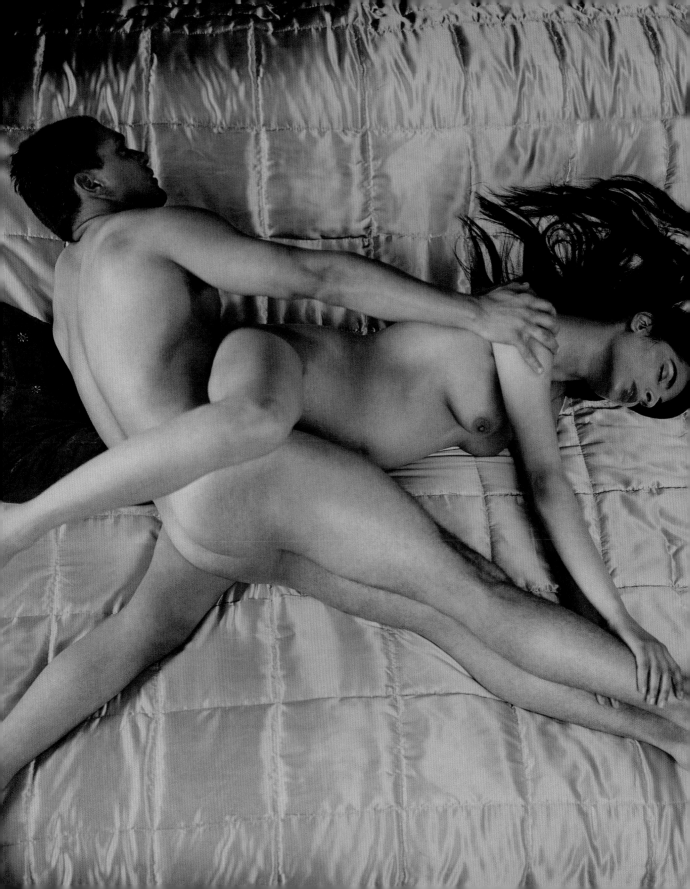

lovers' arch

This is one of those crazy positions that couples fall into when messing around in bed. It probably has more novelty value than pleasurable profit, but the novelty can in itself add to its eroticism.

Before penetration, the man lies at right angles to his lover, puts his legs between hers, then moves his legs around so that she can reach his feet. The unusual angle of entry provides novel sensations for her, as he can touch her from angles she would never otherwise experience. She can also use her hands to stimulate her breasts or clitoris, and stroke her inner thighs. You may find that the creativity of this position makes you feel unexpectedly aroused. And your interest may be sustained by your own erotic fantasies.

During lovemaking, the woman can reach over and massage her lover's buttocks. Some men have such powerful musculature that their buttocks feel quite hard when handled. She might try moving his buttocks in circles underneath the flat of her hand, which will make him feel pleasantly manipulated. If he wants a stronger sensation, she can massage the rest of his body.

By reversing this position, with the man putting his legs outside the woman's, the couple will possibly gain more stimulation from their lovemaking. This reversed position is also perfect for pregnant women, because it avoids putting pressure on her swollen abdomen.

During pregnancy, thanks to increased blood flow and increased vaginal secretions, a woman's vulva may feel particularly engorged, wet, and sensitive—this may lead to more intense orgasms. Her engorged vagina will also hug his penis more tightly during sex, and this can feel great for both lovers.

• THE NINE LEVELS OF AROUSAL

Tao sexology describes a woman's orgasm as a series of rising steps followed by one declining step. Each level of arousal was believed to evoke a certain observable response in the woman. In level one, the woman sighs, breathes heavily, and salivates. In level two, she extends her tongue while kissing. In level three, as her muscles become activated, she grasps him tightly. In level four, she experiences vaginal spasms, and her juices begin to flow. In level five, her joints loosen and she begins to bite. In level six, she undulates, trying to wrap her arms and legs around him. In level seven, she tries to touch her man everywhere. In level eight, her muscles relax, and in level nine, she collapses in a little death, surrenders to her man, and is completely opened up.

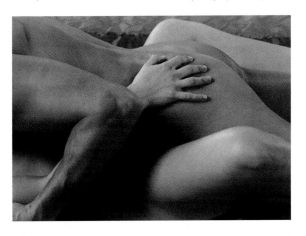

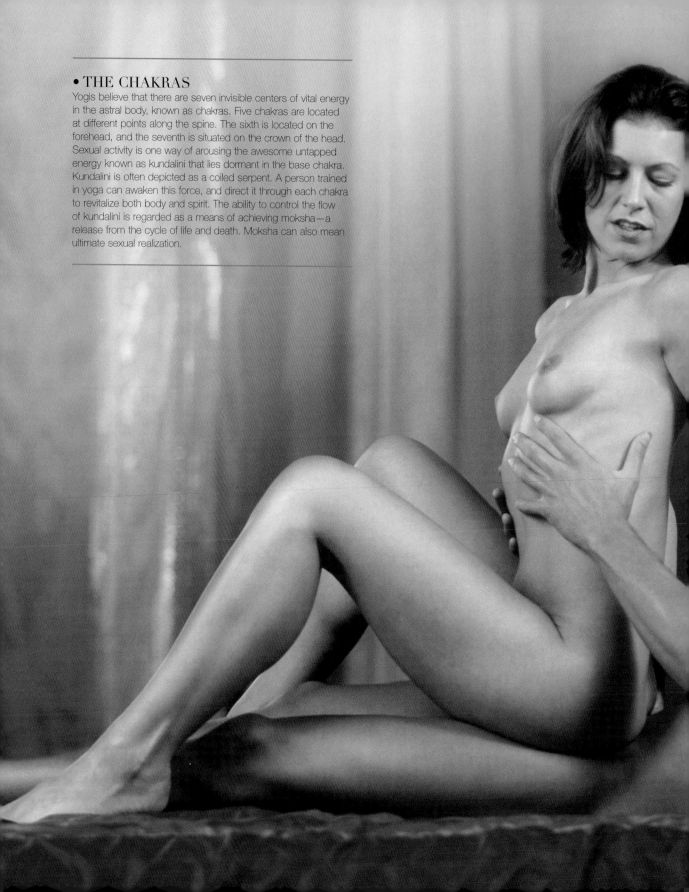

• THE CHAKRAS

Yogis believe that there are seven invisible centers of vital energy in the astral body, known as chakras. Five chakras are located at different points along the spine. The sixth is located on the forehead, and the seventh is situated on the crown of the head. Sexual activity is one way of arousing the awesome untapped energy known as kundalini that lies dormant in the base chakra. Kundalini is often depicted as a coiled serpent. A person trained in yoga can awaken this force, and direct it through each chakra to revitalize both body and spirit. The ability to control the flow of kundalini is regarded as a means of achieving moksha—a release from the cycle of life and death. Moksha can also mean ultimate sexual realization.

the top

Pick up your feet and spin around on his penis—if you dare

This movement requires considerable dexterity, and is only achievable with practice. The idea is that, while sitting astride her partner, the woman raises her legs and swivels around on her man's penis.

This is just about feasible in theory, but spinning without support is difficult, and there is a serious risk of injury to both partners. A less-hazardous, and more stimulating, alternative might be for the woman to use her legs to move herself round. As she performs this maneuver she should take care not to lose her balance, or she may hurt herself and her partner.

If the man is feeling athletic, however, he may also find it exciting to push his woman up and down on his penis in this position and manipulate her so that she swings from side to side, although such movements require a strong man and a very light woman. In general the rewards of this position have more to do with novelty than sexual stimulation. Try this one for the sheer fun of it and to spice up your usual routine, or put it to work more safely in your fantasy life, rather than in the bedroom.

sexy squat

Exercise your muscles by doing squats on your lover's penis

Women-on-top positions usually put her in control to find the stimulation she finds most pleasing. In this position, however, the man reclines on the bed, but her movements are designed to please him.

She sits on top, facing away from her partner, and slips down onto his penis. She braces her feet against the bed or floor, and uses the strength of her thigh muscles to help push her up and down on top of him.

Women: to really turn him on, vary the pace and tempo of your movements. For example, you could use the Tao "Sets of Nine" technique (see page 58), or the "quick, quick, slow" rhythm (see page 87). This will give him a range of stimulation, and create a more sensual experience for you, too. These rhythmic thrusting techniques can work well in most women-on-top positions as well as those controlled by the man.

• HANDS ON

If you want to give your man an extra treat while you're above him in a woman-on-top position, cover one hand with oil or lube and reach down to wrap it round his penis. Use your hand as if it is an extension of your vagina: let it rise and fall as your body rises and falls, so that his penis slips through it as it moves out of your vagina, and receives extra stimulation all along its length. Your hand can grip him much more tightly than your vagina can alone, and he'll find the stimulation intensely exciting.

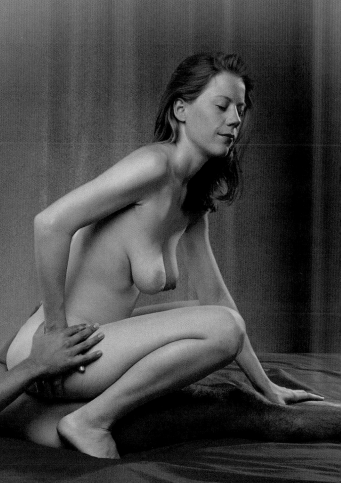

piercing embrace

This intimate and loving embrace also feels sexy and athletic, giving both partners great sensations while still enabling them to kiss, cuddle, and caress each other to orgasm.

Here, the woman sits between her man's knees, so that each lover places the soles of their feet together. After penetration, he moves her back and forth on his penis instead of thrusting from his pelvis. He does this by pulling her toward him, then letting her drop back slightly. Alternatively, she can sit on his feet, which he then moves backward and forward—although he'll need strong legs and arms for this variation. Her role can be passive, or she can place her feet on the ground to help him move her back and forth.

The joy of this position is that these movements are exciting for both partners: he can control the action, and her open legs allow clitoral stimulation.

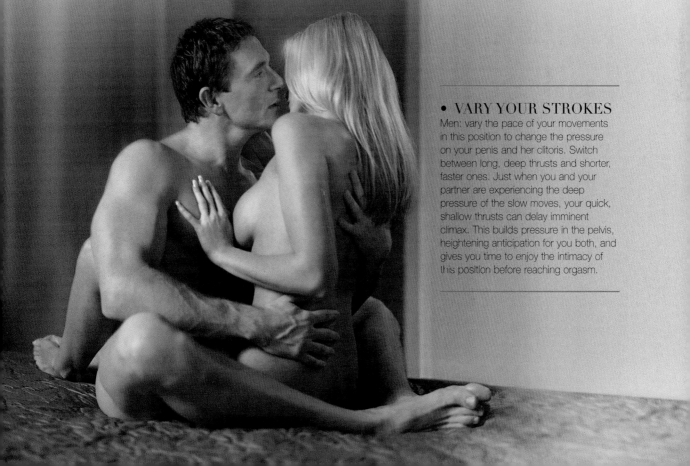

• VARY YOUR STROKES

Men: vary the pace of your movements in this position to change the pressure on your penis and her clitoris. Switch between long, deep thrusts and shorter, faster ones. Just when you and your partner are experiencing the deep pressure of the slow moves, your quick, shallow thrusts can delay imminent climax. This builds pressure in the pelvis, heightening anticipation for you both, and gives you time to enjoy the intimacy of this position before reaching orgasm.

arching back

Find a comfy seat and come together for some X-rated sex

There are some sitting positions that are best achieved with a lot of back support, such as an armchair or sofa. This erotic pose is perfect for impromptu sex, when you can't wait until you get to bed.

The woman controls the angle of the thrusts by leaning back, while he moves her energetically on top of him with his hands. By leaning back, the woman makes herself supremely vulnerable and open to his thrusting.

Although it is usually the partner on top who is the more active, in this position she may find it difficult to move without help. To assist her, the man supports her body with his knees and hands, and controls the pace of lovemaking by lifting her from the waist.

In this position, she can enjoy great stimulation on her clitoris, and many women find the sensation of being manipulated by their man to be deeply arousing. From his comfortable seat, he'll be able to enjoy the sight of her body, and also watch himself thrusting into her—very erotic viewing indeed.

• NEARING HEAVEN

Tantra draws on the belief that the more accomplished your sexual performance becomes, the better you become as a person. Put succinctly, the idea is that you can achieve an ecstatic sense of being through marvelous sex. Each movement and every caress becomes other-worldly; you are nearing "heaven," and the experience becomes a powerful meditation.

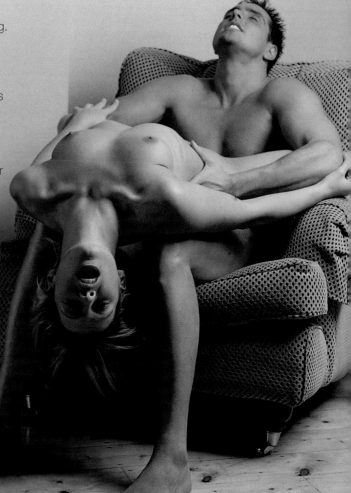

snake trap

Grasp each other's feet and rock to arouse each other

This position is recorded in an ancient sexual manual from the East. The name refers to the fact that, since both lovers grasp each other's feet, there is no escape. His snake is trapped inside her.

The woman sits in her man's lap with her legs to either side of him, while he sits with his legs opened and outstretched, and inserts his penis into her. Both partners lean back, and hold on to each other's feet for support.

This motion gives gentle stimulation, while sitting face to face feels intimate and friendly. This relaxed pose means that either partner can release their foothold from time to time to caress their lover.

Since this position restricts thrusting, it's probably best enjoyed as a physical respite from more vigorous positions, or when you and your partner are tired, or feel like "messing around." This position is unlikely to give either of you dramatic stimulation, but it will offer you a lot of fun and games.

• SITTING POSITIONS
The various sitting positions are not usually intensely stimulating, but they are useful for maintaining a degree of sexual tension over an extended period of time. This kind of slow, tantalizing approach can enable couples to achieve a higher degree of sensual arousal. Stopping during lovemaking to kiss, caress, and stroke each other increases excitement, and this in turn increases the likelihood of mutual or even multiple orgasms.

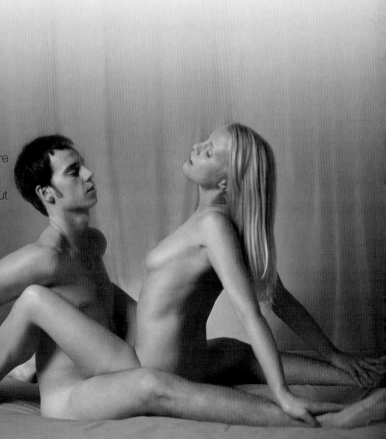

beyond the bedroom

The bedroom isn't the only room that's good for lovemaking. Virtually any room or outside space can be an erotic venue as long as you are assured of privacy. After the bedroom, the bathroom is probably the favorite room for lovemaking. Having sex on the kitchen countertop or on a table can bring new angles, or you could try sex in front of the fire, under the stars, or on the stairs. The erotic possibilities are endless, and variety is a surefire way to add some spontaneity and novelty to your sex life.

Love in the tub

Many couples find that sex follows on naturally from bathing together, and shampooing can be sensual form of foreplay. Start by washing each others' hair, then give a "pelvic shampoo" and wash each others' genitals. Swirl your fingertips in and out of each others' most intimate places.

When you are both aroused, decide whether (and how) you will bring each other to orgasm. Even if your tub isn't big enough to have sex in, you can make love sitting on the edge of the tub, standing up in the shower, or on the floor.

Phone sex

There's nothing very special about a sex chat line, but talking about sex on the phone with your lover is quite different.

If there are things you know they would like done to them, tell them know how you would carry out these actions if you were on the spot.

Describe your self-stimulation as eloquently as possible. Talk your partner through what you're doing, and imagine what he or she is up to. If you use a vibrator or sex toy, tell your partner

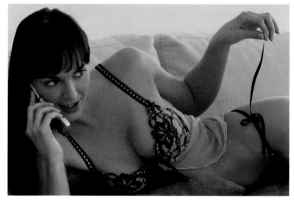

Bathing before sex enhances relaxation and intimacy. If you are feeling stressed out, a warm bath can help to bring on feelings of lazy sensuality.

Before you embark on phone sex, give yourself open-ended time for your call, and make sure that anything you might want to use during sex is within easy reach.

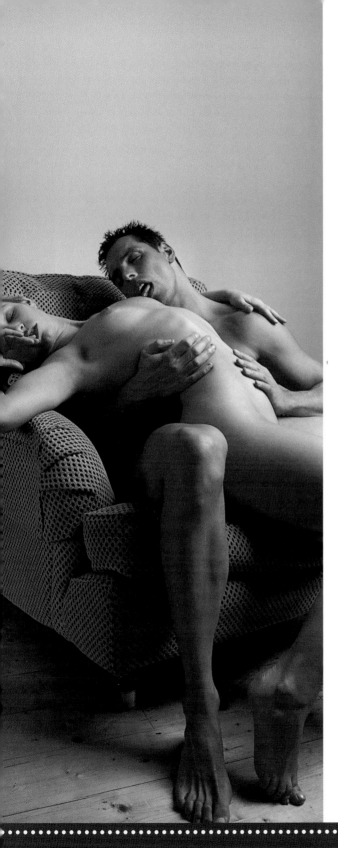

that in your imagination he or she is holding this sex toy, and giving you pleasure. Be explicit and specific in your descriptions. The more detail you go into the better.

Unusual locations

The kitchen is probably most suited for instant passion when you can't wait a moment longer. A table, sink, or counter may be hard, but for sheer novelty, they can't be beaten. And there is always the added thrill you might get caught.

In the living room, any large armchair or deep-sprung sofa is an inviting spot for lovemaking, but the most erotic spot tends to be a thick rug on the floor, preferably stretched out in front of a roaring log fire. Couples might carry out a sensual massage or oral sex here, surrounded by soft music and candlelight.

If you're looking for some new angles for penetration, don't forget to make good use of the stairs on your way up to the bedroom.

It's a beautiful summer's day, and the two of you are lazing in the yard or out on the terrace. What could be more natural than making love in a garden seat or just on the grass. It's a very romantic and different experience?

Just one warning: there are laws in many countries about committing public nuisance or indecency, so only make love where you definitely cannot be observed, or you might find yourself in trouble with the authorities.

Spontaneous lovemaking in an armchair can spice up your love life. Unusual locations give a raw edge to sex, and make it feel exciting and dangerous.

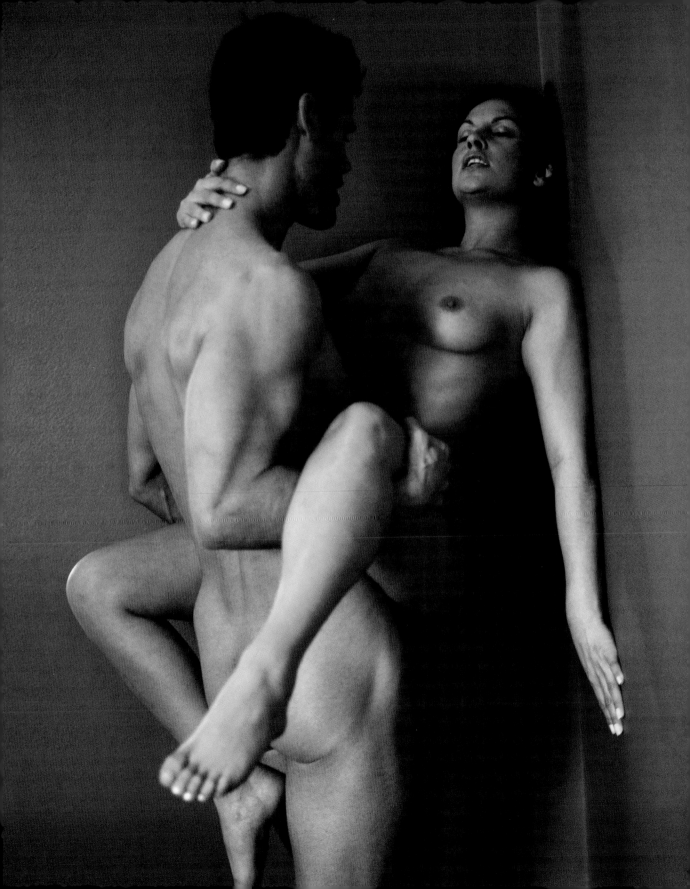

legs entwined upright

Pull him against a wall, wrap your legs around him, and hang on

Humans seem to have an instinctive urge to get as close as possible to their partner during sex. And, for most couples, having sex while standing also feels deliciously forbidden and erotic. This position combines both pleasures.

There is a certain grace in this entwined pose. It feels spontaneous, intimate, and raunchy all at the same time. And this pose enables couples to spice up their sex life without requiring any acrobatic skills.

The woman wraps her crossed legs around her partner, and tightens her leg muscles to draw him closer to her. This energizes her pelvis, and permits a clitoris-stimulating angle of penetration. The man supports her by locking his hands underneath her bottom and leaning her against a wall.

The woman should grip her man with her legs, as if riding a horse, and may need to help his thrusting. It is hard for the man to keep a sensual rhythm going while holding her, so she should push against the wall with her back to give him more support, and help him maintain the thrust of lovemaking.

Often couples start out by making love against a wall, perhaps on the way to the bedroom, but most are glad to fall into bed or the floor to finish off in more comfort. This is one of the ways of keeping your sex life exciting and your attraction fresh. There is nothing quite like falling on each other in such a rush of passion that you don't stop to take off your clothes. Upright sex is also perfect for when you are seized with desire outdoors, although in this case you should always be careful not to do anything against the law.

• SHOWER GAMES

The shower is a natural sex toy: it combines heat, pressure, moisture, and friction all in one device. There are plenty of sensual experiences you and your partner can experiment with and enjoy. Cover each other in liquid soap, and give each other a massage as a sensual precursor to lovemaking. Play around in the shower, and use the water jets on an alternate pleasure/punishment basis. Pleasure is warm water directed at the genitals; punishment is a blast of cold water on the back. Men: see if you can masturbate her to orgasm using only the jets of water from the showerhead. Women: surprise him with oral sex.

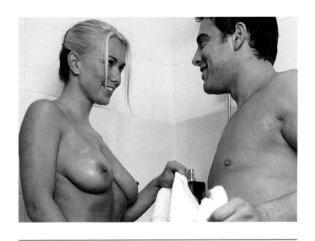

wheelbarrow in the air

Find a chair, grab your lover, and test your muscles to the max

This position is an exciting and athletic experience, and useful as a follow-up to a more conventional seated or kneeling position when one or both of you want to heat up your lovemaking.

The woman kneels on the floor and grabs on to a chair, and her partner lifts her by her thighs, spreads her legs, and penetrates her. The man is firmly in control of the thrusting action. This one is definitely not for the frail, or anyone with a bad back. In general, you should avoid holding this position for more than a few thrusts because it might cause her an injury.

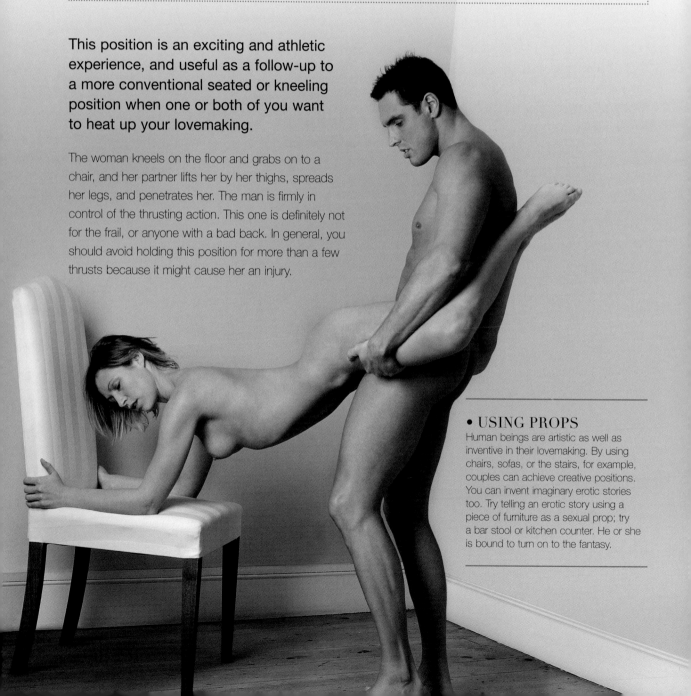

• USING PROPS

Human beings are artistic as well as inventive in their lovemaking. By using chairs, sofas, or the stairs, for example, couples can achieve creative positions. You can invent imaginary erotic stories too. Try telling an erotic story using a piece of furniture as a sexual prop; try a bar stool or kitchen counter. He or she is bound to turn on to the fantasy.

bottoms up

Defy gravity in this playful, upside-down, bottom-tingling pose

Size really does matter in this crazy pose. It is probably only possible if the man has a long or curved penis, but may appeal to couples with a sense of adventure or those looking for a head rush.

The man and woman start in a standing position, then bend over so their buttocks are touching, and support their weight by putting their hands on the floor. Unless the man and woman are the same height, her feet will need to be propped up as high as possible to give her man a sporting chance of success.

To penetrate her, he reaches down and pushes his penis back between his thighs to aim at her vagina, and uses shallow, forcible thrusts without withdrawing his penis from her.

The position may prove too difficult for many couples to achieve successfully, and neither partner will enjoy great stimulation, but so what? You can fall over laughing or collapse into giggles together as you strive to give each other pleasure. And you may find it a titillating and fun prelude to more sensual, and rewarding, lovemaking positions.

• NAMING THE PARTS

The writers of the many Chinese Taoist pillow books, like their Indian and Arabian counterparts, took much inspiration from nature when describing sexual matters, and gave evocative descriptions of the male and female genitals. For example, the male sexual organ was given names such as "jade stem," "male stalk," "red bird," and "heavenly dragon pillar." Some of the poetic names for the female sexual organ included "coral gate," "jade gate," "open peony blossom," "receptive vase," and "jade step" (clitoris).

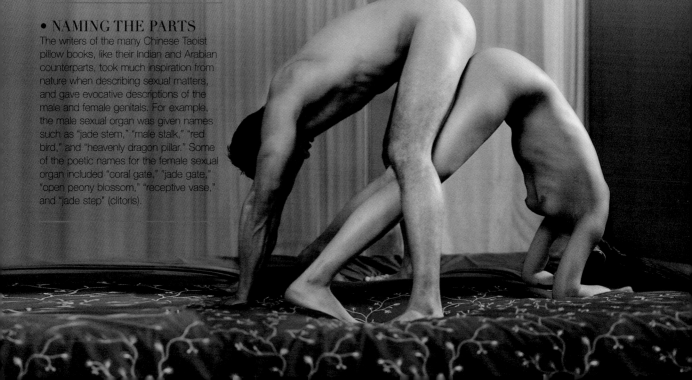

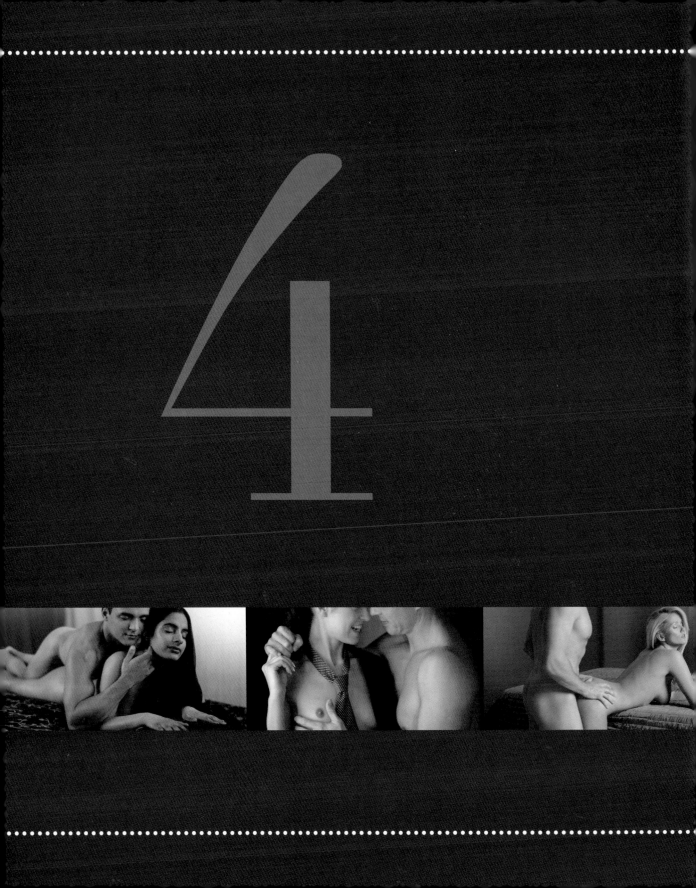

Sex Games and Adventures

Fantasy and games are an entirely natural part of a legitimate sex life. Thousands of men and women secretly fantasize as a way of reaching and enhancing climax. The mind plays an essential role in how both men and women experience desire, excitement, and orgasm. This chapter provides a vivid insight into some of the most common male and female fantasies, for you and your partner to consider working into your sex life.

Indulge in some light bondage in the Package or the Racing Horse. Dominate your lover with spanks and strokes in Taming the Tiger. Or submit completely to your lover's will in Role-reversal. Foster your erotic fantasies in the Fantasy Duet, and discover how to enter the forbidden zones of your lover's body with anal play.

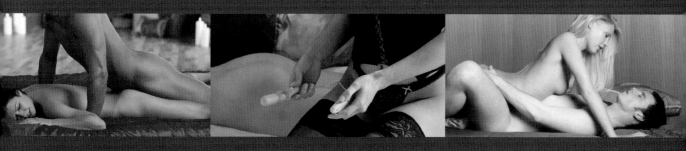

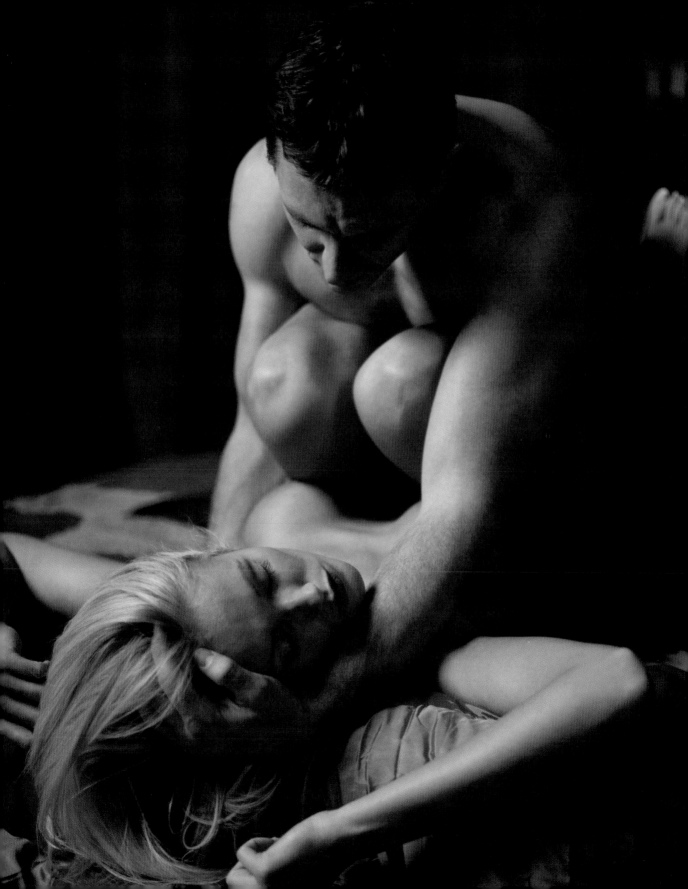

the package

Make her helpless with desire by taking charge of her pleasure

Many couples love submission and domination (S&D) games—they enjoy role-playing and letting their deepest sexual fantasies come to life.

This position has an air of S&D about it, as the woman is physically confined and the man is in control. She lies on her back with her legs close to her body and her knees resting on her partner's chest. His knees are positioned outside her thighs, and he puts one hand under her buttocks to lift her slightly as he enters her.

After he has penetrated, the man can support her on his thighs so that his hands are free to roam across her body. If she finds herself turned on by lack of control and feelings of helplessness, she may find this position extremely arousing mentally, although physically it may not offer much stimulation.

This position is the perfect introduction to S&D games, particularly if she is eager to join him in a bondage game, but unwilling to be tied up. It shows that sexual role-play can be as simple as the seducer having his wicked way with the virgin. To follow up, you might try a slave-and-sultan scenario where the sultan demands helpless passivity from his harem of concubines.

Try fantasies in turn, starting with gentle scenarios and building up slowly to the stronger ones. This allows you to make sure you both enjoy the experience, and to back out if you don't.

Take turns at being dominant or submissive. Good sex generally means that anything goes; in other words, "Whatever you want to do (within reason) is OK by me if I love and trust you." Acting out each other's sexual fantasies should serve ultimately to strengthen your bond of intimacy and trust with your lover.

• S&D GAMES

The list of S&D role-plays is endless: master and servant, drill sergeant and foot soldier, professor and student, dominatrix and client. But whatever the scenario, there are always certain aims in these games. If you are in charge, your aim will be to create pleasurable anticipation in your partner. The submissive partner should enjoy relinquishing power, and revel in their lack of responsibility. In turn, the dominating partner will gain reassurance that their behaviour is acceptable and, if they lead the game well, will feel a sense of strength. The games should promote trust and intimacy, and be arousing to both parties. Punishments for disobedience play a part, and might include light spanking, genital exposure, and vaginal or anal penetration.

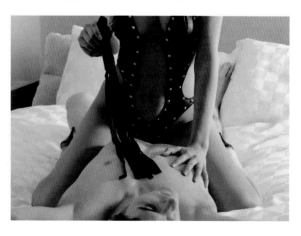

see-saw

Get in rhythm with him and set a climax-triggering pace

Despite its man-on-top appearance, the woman dominates in this position, since by tensing or relaxing her legs she controls the depth and rhythm of thrusting.

She lies with her legs parted while he kneels between her legs. She then lifts her knees to squeeze her lover around his waist and reaches back to grasp the headboard for support.

Once he has penetrated her, the man leans forward to grasp her hands. Although movement for both partners is limited, the man must respond to her rhythm, as he is reliant on the tension in her legs to give him something to push against. Supporting themselves against the headboard, the lovers move back and forth in a seesaw motion, and the action of pulling and pushing against the bed in this way can bring them both a thrilling sense of urgency.

• FANTASIZING
Men are often more prone to sexual fantasy than women, but fantasy is an important part of sexuality in both sexes. A fantasy can help build excitement, heighten your orgasm, and can provide a solution for women who experience difficulty climaxing. Many women are uncomfortable with sexual fantasy and devise reasons for keeping their minds "pure," but allowing yourself to let go can greatly improve your enjoyment of sex.

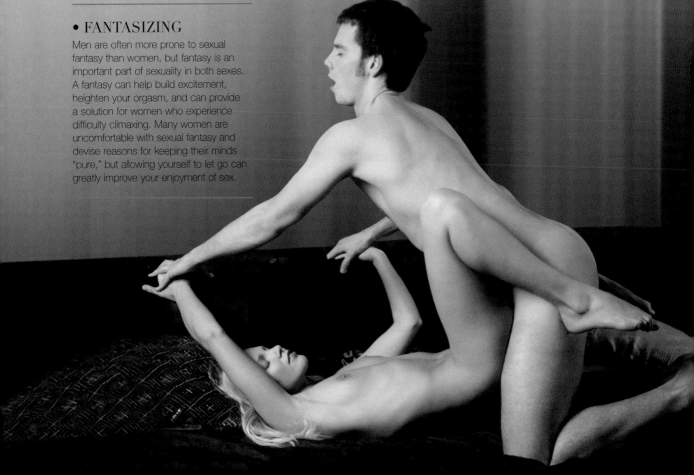

taming the tiger

Stroke, spank, or both—she chooses in this provocative pose

The woman's pose resembles that of a tigress during congress. Most men love the eroticism of watching their woman's buttocks move as they thrust into her.

This rear-entry position calls for the man to kneel as he thrusts into his woman from behind. He can draw her to him by placing his hands on her waist, and she can raise or lower her body to suit her partner's height. This also means that she can change the angle of penetration to enjoy maximum stimulation.

Women: encourage your man to stimulate your clitoris by asking him to reach between your legs and stroke you as he thrusts. For extra stimulation, get him to use a fingertip clitoral vibrator.

Men: if you want to raise the sexual tension, you can – with her permission—give your lover a spank on the bottom, clapping the palm of your hand smartly on the fleshy part of her buttock. After a spank, rub her buttocks to take away the sting. Or you can replace spanking with gentle stroking if she prefers.

• SPANKING AND STROKING

Spanking can be very sexy for both partners. First, it gives a novel physical sensation—it makes the skin feel hot and tingly. Second, spanking offers a psychological thrill. The message it sends is: "I'm in charge and I want you to know it." Spanking can also be used as punishment in S&D and role-play games. To spank without hurting, use the flat of your hand not your fingers. Don't strike repeatedly in the same place, and never spank on bony areas. Fleshy areas like the buttocks are the best. If your ministrations cause your partner real pain, then you should stop.

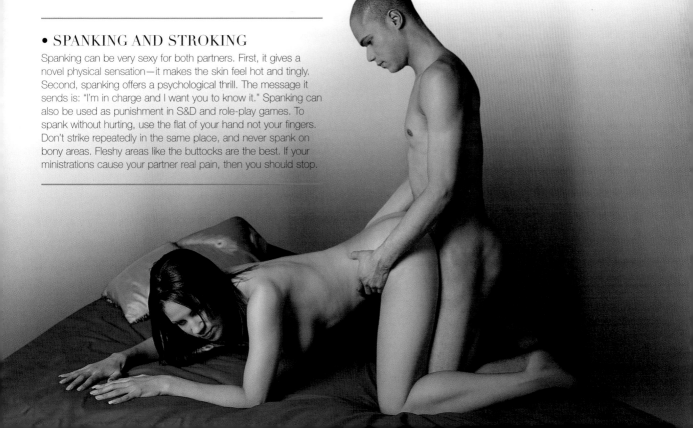

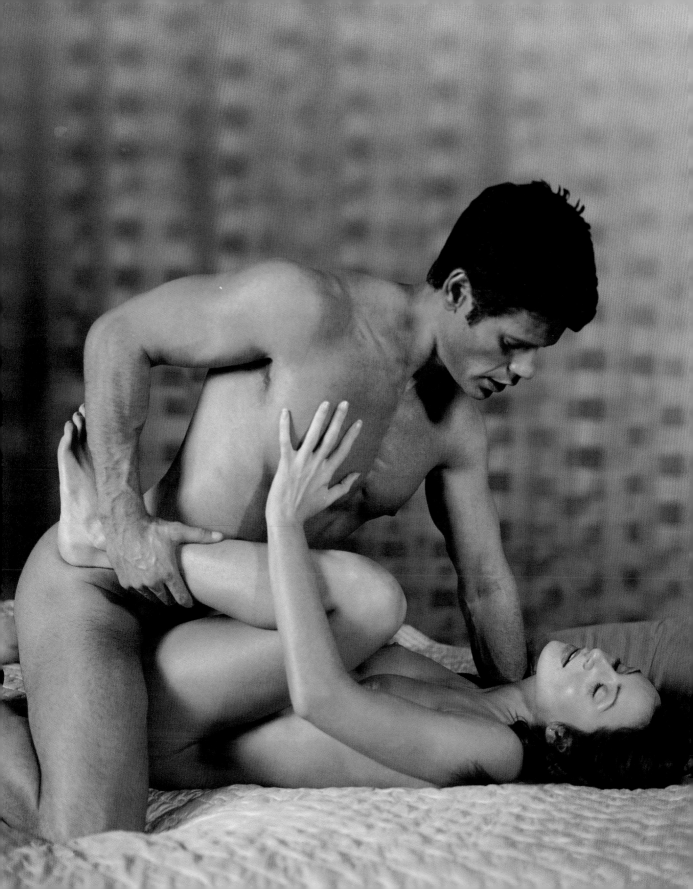

racing horse

Grasp her ankle and draw her close for galloping thrills

In this position, the woman's hand and knee movements are controlled by her man, and resemble the motion of a horse's legs crossing over as it gallops.

There are distinct undertones of bondage in this position, due to the way the man holds his lover's ankle and locks her leg into position. As with "the package" (see pages 144–145), couples might like to try this position as a gentle introduction to the many delights of S&D games.

The woman lies on her back and bends her left knee, while the man kneels in front of her and leans over her. He steadies himself by placing his left hand just by her right shoulder, clasps her left ankle with his right hand and, drawing her close, penetrates her. He then thrusts fast to gain the sensation of galloping.

The woman can, if she wishes, clasp her man's right hand so that she rocks in time with his "galloping" movements. Some women find this easier if both legs are bent instead of just one, which allows deeper penetration and more clitoral stimulation.

This is a very restricting position for her, as she must submit her body completely to her lover. If this is part of an S&D role-play, agree on a code word before starting any games. Part of the thrill of such games comes from pretended unwillingness on the part of

one partner, and you might agree beforehand that simply saying "Stop it" will be part of the game. But the use of a code word means you really do want to stop. Always respect your partner's wishes. If you have the mildest suspicion that your partner will not play by the rules, don't even consider starting this type of activity.

• THE ATTRACTIONS OF BONDAGE

Bondage is simply the tying up of one partner during sex to restrict his or her movement. The dominant partner can then tease their restrained lover into submission. Some people need to feel securely contained, because they find it hard to "let go" enough to enjoy sexuality. If they are rendered helpless, there is nothing they can do to prevent erotic stimulation; the constraint somehow makes it okay to experience pleasure. The variety of bondage props is enormous, from silken scarves, ties, and haberdashery-style ropes, to commercial bondage kits consisting of specially designed couches which you can adjust to gain the perfect angle of penetration, "swings" to strap yourself into, and even sets of "love stirrups" to wear during sex.

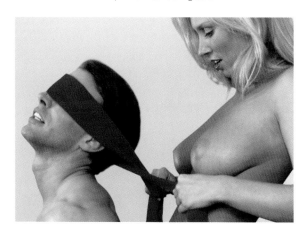

sex games

Many couples love playing games in the bedroom, and sharing a fantasy is the best sort of spontaneous sex game. There are many ways to act out the porn movies of your imagination: you can wear costumes or masks, use props, decorate your bedroom in erotic style, or rely on imagination, role-play, and story telling. Discuss your fantasies with your lover; finding out what they dislike or are unsure of will help establish the ground rules for game playing. Be honest, but also non-judgmental.

Acting out a fantasy

The beauty of sexual intimacy is that you can re-visit activities that you last considered during childhood, such as playing imaginary roles.

There are a number of fantasy scenarios that you and your partner can enjoy together, such as virgin and pirate, professor and pupil, nurse and patient, slave and mistress. Take turns playing the submissive or dominant role.

Fantasy visuals

Visual stimulation is very important to a man's arousal—his sex drive can be easily awakened by the sight of a female stripping.

Before you begin your striptease, ensure that the lighting is soft and moody and the room is warm. If you are wearing stockings and heels, consider leaving them on for as long as possible, and during any sex that follows.

Remember to enjoy the experience—stripping isn't just for your lover, it's also a chance to show off your sexuality and enjoy the attention.

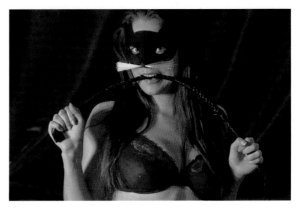

Spanking and light caning can accelerate desire of both giver and receiver, particularly when used as part of a punishment/reward game for good or bad behavior.

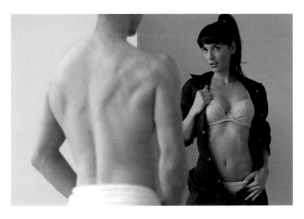

If you're stripping for your partner, make sure that the clothes you are taking off are sexy, such as seductive underwear—this will add to the sensual effect.

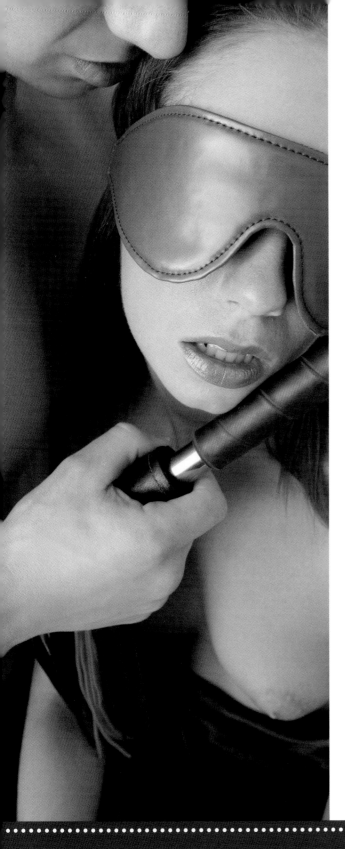

Mirrors placed at strategic points around your bedroom and home can be used for special scenarios of exhibitionism and voyeurism. These always add a certain frisson to sexual proceedings, and they have the advantage of not seeming to be premeditated. Your sexual "acting" in front of them can therefore evolve completely naturally without embarrassment or "stage fright."

Blindfolds and restraints

Most S&D games involve one partner wearing restraints and/or a blindfold. This is because the aim of many S&D games is to stir your partner's X-rated imagination. To frustrate your partner by tantalizing and teasing can paradoxically lead to greater satisfaction. Not being able to have what you desire arouses many people, and this increases the degree of sexual turn-on.

A blindfold also creates a sense of helplessness and vulnerability. You don't know where you are when you wear it, and you have no idea what obstacles you might be facing. For comfort, use a soft material such as a silk scarf, or a black velvet eye mask. Make sure that you don't tie the blindfold too tightly, but don't leave it too loose unless partial sight is part of a game.

Unless you know that your partner is into really serious bondage, it's best to use restraints made of soft fabrics, such as a silk tie, or silky cords. Alternatively, most of the sex-toy manufacturers sell "safe" handcuffs, specially designed for the purpose of sex-play.

The thrill of power games comes from establishing your dominance or your vulnerability, so couples might want to spend a whole evening or day playing these games.

thoughts of bondage

Dominate your man in this erotic pose that puts her in charge

This sexy woman-on-top position is ideal for putting her in control of penetration. The slow up-and-down movements give her plenty of erotic stimulation to help her gradually reach climax.

She sits on her lover's hips, inserts his penis into her vagina, and leans back with her hands braced on his legs. She then flexes her legs to move her hips slowly up and down on his penis. By leaning back, she can ensure that his penis stimulates her G-spot, with the added bonus that he can manually stimulate her clitoris at the same time. If her legs begin to tire with the up-and-down movements, he can reach forward to hold her hips and help her rise and fall.

The role-reversal position may serve to heighten each partner's erotic desires. The tantalizing movement of her body, with her knees jutting high, is a pleasure for him to watch, although he may feel vulnerable, especially since she can injure his penis by leaning back too far or allowing it to slip out.

• THE EROTIC INVENTOR FANTASY

Tell your lover that you've invented some new sex toys and you need a subject to test them on. Do this in an entirely clinical manner—you might even wear a white coat. Having invested in a collection of toys, begin the testing. Write down his or her comments on a pleasure scale of one to ten. When you have worked your way through the toys, select the one that rated highest, and put the star invention to full use.

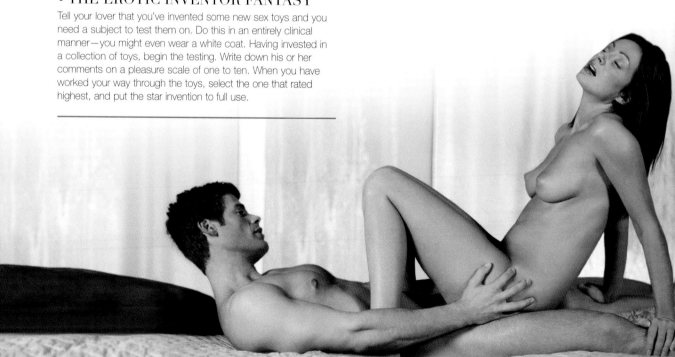

hands down

Bend over and wiggle your bottom to drive him wild with desire

This is an unusual sex position, involving rear-entry sex where both parties are standing, but it is perfect for making love in the bathtub or shower.

In this position, the man gets an erotic view of his woman's buttocks and genitals as she stretches down and touches the ground with her hands. He penetrates and thrusts from behind her while holding on to her hips. The woman can alter his angle of penetration by bending her knees slightly.

She will be unable to make any real movements of her own, so the man must hold his partner firmly with both hands on her hips and pull and let go rhythmically to achieve stimulation. As well as being effective, this pose is an exercise in balance.

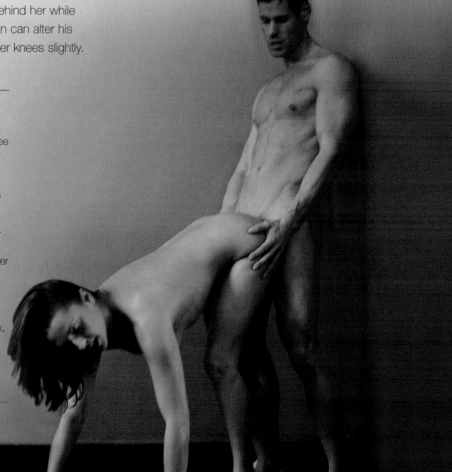

• MALE MULTIPLES

Male multiple orgasms are not a myth, but achieving them requires a high degree of muscle control. To achieve a multiple orgasm, you must be able to block the flow of ejaculate by constricting the muscles in your penis. Various exercises can help with this. Learn testicle control by standing with your feet apart and pulling your testicle muscles toward your lower abdomen. Repeat this as often as possible, but stop if you feel pain. Another way is to give yourself an erection and train yourself to maintain it for as long as possible. Finally, arouse yourself slowly, building up a pitch of excitement over a long time. When you feel about to climax, clench your pelvic-floor muscles (see page 124) and attempt to slow down, or even stop, your ejaculation. If you succeed, you can try for another climax.

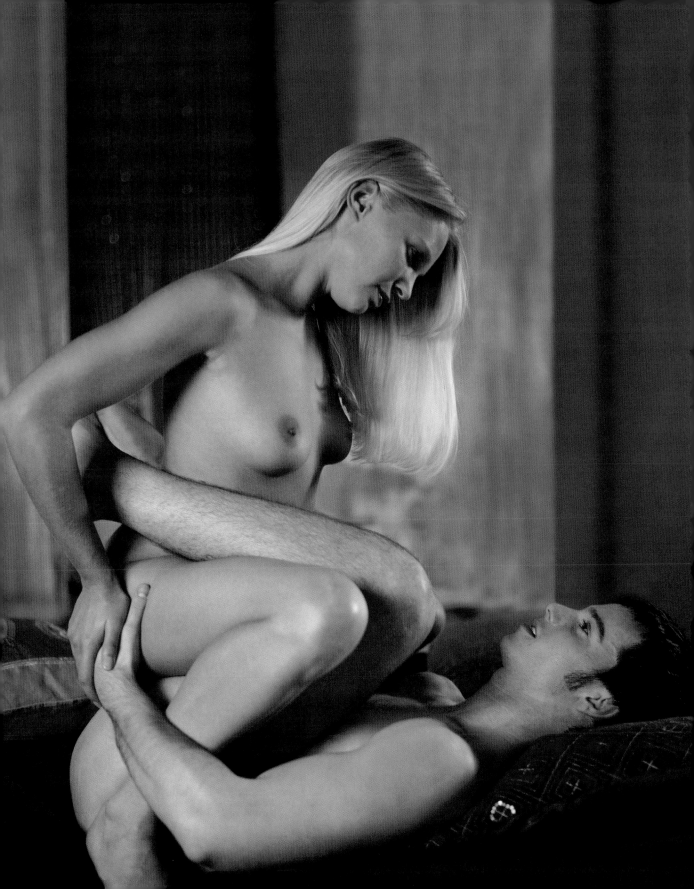

role-reversal

Spice up your sex life by changing places for the night

Who is in charge in your relationship? If one of you always plays the sexual predator while the other tends to take a more passive role, you might both enjoy swapping places for the night.

For men, having sex in a submissive position can heighten their erotic thoughts as well as physical sensations. Likewise, women may find that they are turned on by the sexual power of being in charge, and the thought of their man being vulnerable and receptive to their sexual wishes.

Here, the man lies with a large cushion under his shoulders and draws his knees up to form a V-shape. She faces him, lowers herself down between his thighs, and inserts his penis into her vagina.

In the advanced version, shown here, the man pulls his knees up toward his shoulders so his lover can sit astride his thighs and "ride" him. She needs to push herself up and down on his erect penis by bending her knees. The movement is very like doing knee-bends while skiing—fitness as you frolic.

She is in charge in this position, and her man will feel an erotic frisson from being made love to. He can also enjoy watching and stroking her body. She'll enjoy great stimulation from her up-and-down movements, and can move his hands to her clitoris to show him

where she wants to be stroked. The downside is that this position requires the woman to have strong legs, and the muscle strain and physical effort mean that she may not be able to continue for long. But, while her legs hold out, she can enjoy the feeling of being in control and watching her partner's reactions.

• CROSS-DRESSING FOR HIM

For men, dressing up as the opposite sex can help liberate their softer, more feminine side. You might be surprised by how the experience of swapping genders affects what you do, say, and how you have sex. Get into the role by dressing in a skirt and blouse (or a dress)—your lover's if they will fit you. Make sure you are clean-shaven and apply moisturizer and foundation to your skin. Follow this with mascara on your eyelashes and a coat of lipstick on your lips. Practice walking in high heels—take much smaller steps than you would do normally. Speed up your body movements, and use your hands to express your thoughts and feelings. Deliberately heighten your voice so that it hits an upper register. Be playful and have fun in your new role.

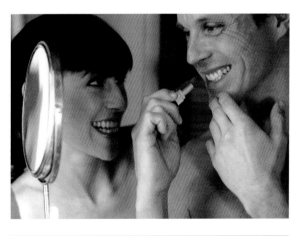

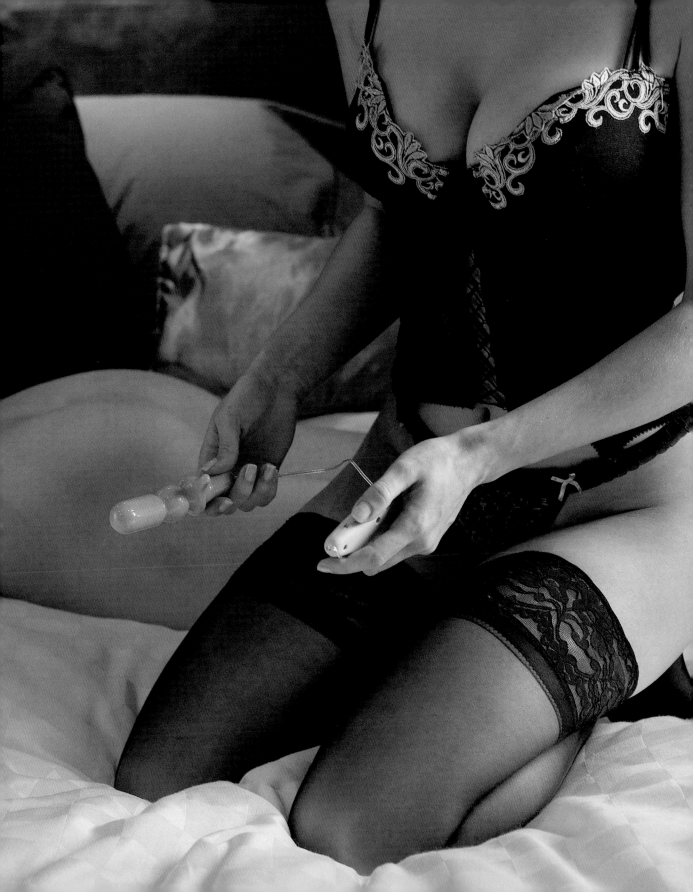

p-spot pleasure

Swap over, it's time to explore his rosebud

Although not all men—or women—are comfortable with the idea, stimulation inside his anus can be a source of great pleasure for him. In fact, it is one of the best-kept sexual secrets of all time.

Don't feel obliged to try prostate massage—you must both make a completely free choice to explore this technique. If you are interested, however, start by stroking the highly sensitive entrance to his anal passage. Very short fingernails are a prerequisite, and because the anal area has no natural lubrication you will need to apply a good gooey lubricant.

Begin by massaging the outer region of the anus. Using a gentle pressure, run a well-lubricated finger around the outside of the "rosebud." Next, insert a finger slightly and gently run it around the inside of the anus. Push softly against the outer entrance to stretch him as you do this. Then slide a slightly curved finger in and out, moving from the front to the back of his body. Slide your finger in and out by about an inch (2cm) without withdrawing it completely.

The P-spot (prostate gland) is located on the uppermost side at the far end of the anal passage, at approximately the 12 o'clock position. Your finger, however, may not be long enough to reach it, in which case try an anal toy (see page 165). When his "rosebud" has relaxed, try stroking the P-spot with a slightly curved finger as if beckoning, over and over

again. It's the softness of a finger pad that's needed here. If you can sustain this movement, it's highly likely to make him wild with pleasure, and he may reach orgasm quickly. His anal passage will contract forcefully as he climaxes, so wait until it has relaxed before gently withdrawing your finger.

• THE P-SPOT
The P-spot can be considered to be the male equivalent of the female G-spot. "P" stands for "prostate," the gland which produces seminal fluid. The gland itself is located at the top of the anal passage on the upper side, nearest his belly. Feel around for a slight bump. The entire anal region is laden with sensitive nerve endings, and the P-spot is the most dynamic area. This hidden pleasure zone tends to be overlooked by both sexes, perhaps because penetration of the male is considered feminizing and taboo. This is a pity because massage of the prostate alone can bring a man to orgasm. If your partner enjoys manual stimulation of the area, you may want to try P-spot sex toys (see page 165) to add further excitement.

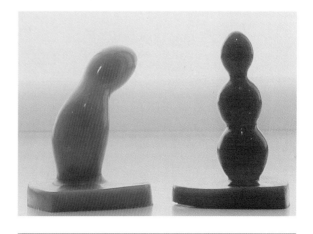

erotic spoons

Cozy up in spoons, then go beyond conventional lovemaking

Many people, both men and women, find anal intercourse extremely sensual and exciting. The anus is full of sensitive nerve endings which feel wonderful when stimulated by a fingertip or a penis.

To enjoy anal intercourse, it is vital that the woman is relaxed and the man proceeds slowly. The key is to use plenty of lubricant and begin slowly by stretching her anus using finger massage.

Start by stroking her perineum, then use a well-lubricated finger to rim around her anus. Make sure your partner is enjoying the experience before proceeding to slip one, then two fingers into her anus.

If she allows him to penetrate her, he should insert his penis by degrees and very gently. The advantage of this position is that he can see whether or not she is enjoying herself. For added protection, use an extra-strong condom designed specifically for anal sex.

• HOT BOT SPOTS

The buttocks are an erogenous zone, and using your finger to probe and stretch adds a sensual build-up to anal sex. When using your fingers (men and women) in anal play, think of the anus as a clock, with the 12 o'clock position closest to the vagina or testicles. The most erogenous points are usually at 10 and 2 o'clock. When exploring the anal area, it is vital to probe gently.

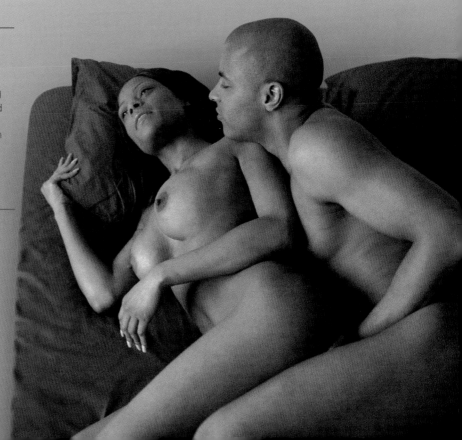

pleasure seat

Get comfortable on his lap, and take control of the action

If you and your partner both enjoy anal sex, you may want to try out this more advanced version, in which the woman sits on her partner's penis to allow him to penetrate her deeply.

Here, the man sits on a chair or the edge of the bed, and the woman sits on his lap. He should make sure that her anal passage is well lubricated and sufficiently

stretched before penetration to avoid discomfort, perhaps by manual massage or analingus (oral stimulation of the anus).

The woman takes control of penetration, and by moving up and down on his penis can enjoy gentle thrusting. Her man can support her by helping to lift her up and down. He can finger her clitoris at the same time to help bring her to climax.

• NATURAL SEX

Many heterosexuals as well as homosexuals find anal sex completely natural and spontaneously sensual. Many women are profoundly turned on by a combination of anal penetration (or fingering) and clitoral stimulation. However, it is vital to ensure that you are both scrupulously clean. Always use a condom for anal sex, and never go from anal to vaginal sex without washing.

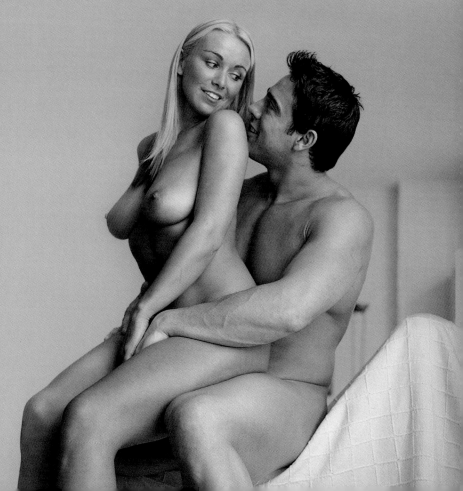

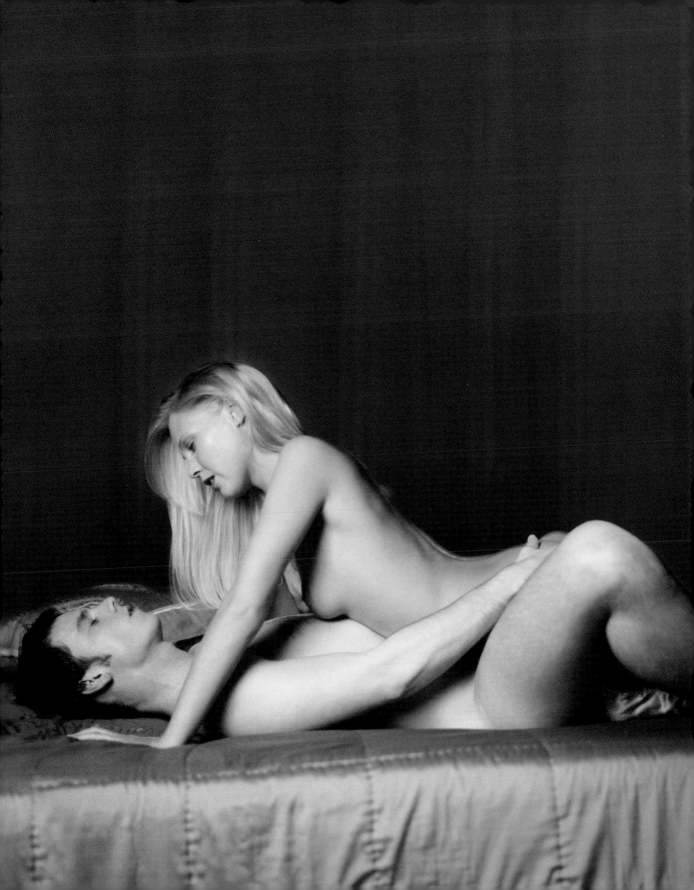

Push-up

When a heterosexual woman puts on a man's clothes and acts like a man, she gets an insight into what it's like to be a man. And this sense of "masculinity" may lend power to her everyday behavior.

In the "push-up" she takes the male role, and her on-top thrusting motions require him to submit to her for the duration. You don't have to change into men's clothes to enjoy this position, unless you want to.

The man lies on his back with his legs open and a cushion resting between his thighs. She lies on top of him to enable him to penetrate her, then closes her legs. Her movements in this position are like a sophisticated version of a push-up, in which she levers herself up and down on top of him while her vagina and thighs tightly grip his penis.

By varying the angle of thrust slightly, she can ensure that her clitoris is stimulated. She should move her pelvis close up against her partner's to enable this to happen. He should pull her buttocks firmly toward him so that you both enjoy deeper penetration.

Women might be surprised how turned on they get by this role reversal position. The feeling of sexual power can be exhilarating, and it may make your man feel more vulnerable and receptive—two qualities that don't always come easily to men. This is a particularly excellent lovemaking position for an older man and his younger partner, because it gives the penis the extra stimulation that many older men need in order to reach climax. But for any couple, this position means that he gets the opportunity to lie back, relinquish control, and simply enjoy being made love to by his woman.

• BE A DRAG KING

Women: try dressing in your lover's shirts and pants, or wear clothes that have a masculine edge to them, such as a pin-striped suit. Tie or push your hair back off your face, and leave your face completely free of make-up. Try to smell like a man too. Whatever scent you associate with masculinity— aftershave or fresh sweat, for example—wear it with pride. Change your posture and body language. Sit with your legs wide apart rather than crossing them. Place your feet flat on the ground. When you stand up, take your time and lean forward before straightening up. When walking, don't wiggle your hips or bottom, and make your strides longer than usual. Let your voice drop to its lowest natural pitch and enjoy your "masculinity."

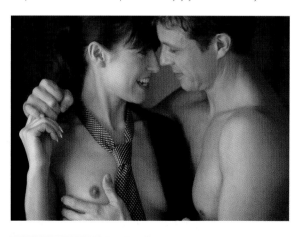

fantasy duet

Foster erotic fantasies, and slip into a sensual world of your own

Making love in this rather impersonal fashion allows both partners to have erotic fantasies about enjoying sex elsewhere, or by unconventional means, or even with other people.

In a long-term partnership, desire can sometimes wane as familiarity grows. In this case, it can be useful to employ fantasies during lovemaking to help re-ignite sexual excitement between you.

In this "duet," the man lies on his back, ideally with his head propped up with a cushion so that he can get a pleasing view of his woman's buttocks as she rises and falls above him. She sits astride him with her legs between his, and leans forward.

The woman may look down so that she can see the action of penetration, or close her eyes and enter a fantasy world. Her balance is best maintained by leaning forward slightly during lovemaking.

• EXPLORING TABOOS

The idea of a fantasy taboo is a contradiction in terms. After all, the whole point of a fantasy is that it is something your brain produces, virtually in spite of yourself. We may dream of experiencing passion with someone of the same sex, or with a famous movie star. We may even dream of sex with someone "forbidden," such as a relative or a best-friend's partner, or of being taken by—or taking—someone unwillingly. Our dreams, however, do not necessarily mean that we want to make the fantasy a reality: it is the idea that turns us on.

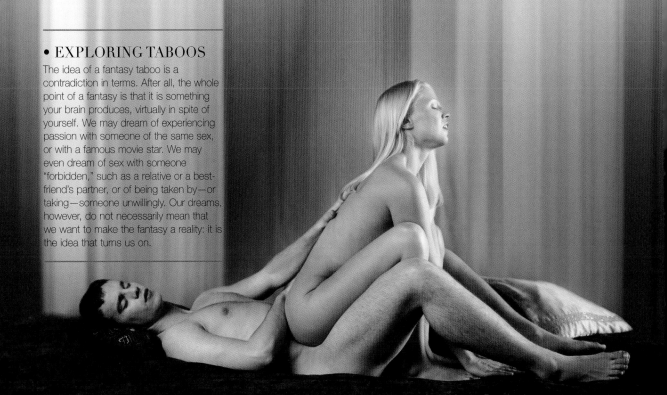

keeping your balance

Grab onto a chair to raise the erotic temperature

Some of the best sex is spontaneous, when couples are overcome with passion and feel an urgent desire for immediate gratification, without waiting to go to bed.

In this position, the woman kneels on a chair and her partner penetrates her from behind. Holding on to the back of the chair will help her keep her balance.

The sensation of being nude in the living room or kitchen can feel deliciously forbidden, so a degree of discomfort can be forgotten in the throes of passion. In the back of the mind, the additional thought of being discovered can add a special "frisson" to lovemaking.

Experiment with using other props for your lovemaking. The edge of a sofa can work just as well as a chair for intercourse in kneeling positions. Sex on the edge of a kitchen table may not be entirely satisfactory, because

kitchen tables are hard and cold and lovers don't respond well to discomfort, but often it is the idea of what you are doing and where you are doing it that makes impromptu sex so exciting.

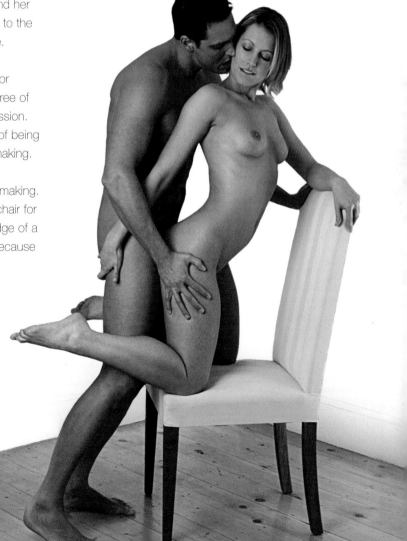

• SEXUAL PATTERNS

Many couples tend to follow a sexual pattern or routine with a partner, favoring positions or techniques that they have both become comfortable with and that they know will give them satisfaction. However, most of us enjoy novelty. To spice up your love life, experiment with a few alternative positions once in a while. Try sex while kneeling or standing to add something new to your usual routine and rekindle your desires.

sex toys

The best sex often uses props to extend and enhance the action. If straight sex is your favorite, then a vibrator will add to the excitement. If something darker gets your pulse racing, look to blindfolds, restraints, and a variety of sex toys to extend your sensual experience. A well-stocked toy box might include vibrators (anal and vaginal), dildos, cock rings, anal wands, butt plugs, lube, a blindfold, a fur mitt, feathers, a paddle, silken cords or "safe" handcuffs, edible body paint, face masks, and disguises.

Twice the fun

Double-pleasure vibrators consist of two stimulating devices: one large and penis-shaped for vaginal penetration; the second is small and curved for anal stimulation. A double-ended dildo is designed so that one end can be inserted into each of the woman's orifices, and so maximize her stimulation.

Silicone balls are weighted spheres designed to slip into the vagina for pleasure alone or during intercourse. They can also be used to tone a woman's vaginal muscles.

Clitoral and G-spot joy

A vibrator gives a woman an extra blast of clitoral stimulation, and are perfect for solo masturbation. The problem with most vibrators, however, is that their phallic shape makes them difficult to wedge between you and your partner when you have sex.

One solution is to use a clitoral vibrator that is designed to be worn on the man's penis; the other is to use a special, ergonomically designed vibrator that curves around the woman's pubic bone and vibrates against her clitoris.

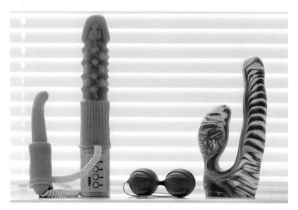

Double-pleasure vibrators, silicone balls, and double dildos are intended for mutual stimulation, and can be used by couples to gain a number of different sensations.

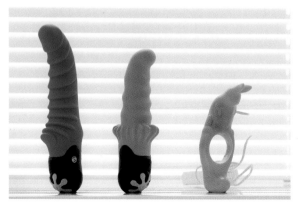

Silicone vibrators tend to be the most penis-like, while three-in-one vibrators (right) can be slipped over the man's penis, and the "rabbit ears" stimulate the clitoris.

If a woman enjoys G-spot stimulation, but both partners finds it difficult to get their fingers in the right place, a vibrator with a curved tip can help. Move the vibrator up and down the front wall of her vagina to find the place that yields the most intense sensations. The better-quality vibrators pulsate instead of vibrate, and some do both. If she prefers static pressure on her G-spot, try a dildo with a curved tip.

Toys for boys

Many women find that their fingers are too short to reach as far as his P-spot. This is where sex toys make a spectacular addition. P-spot vibrators are slimmer than vaginal cigar-shaped ones; they bulge slightly in the middle, and have a small hilt at the end. The slimness is to make anal penetration easy, the bulge is to hold the vibrator in place once it has moved up the anus, and the hilt is to ensure that it doesn't travel too far inside. The newest varieties work with pulsation, not just vibration, which is especially stimulating for the P-spot.

Anal beads are also very popular, and comprise a string of connected plastic spheres. Once the beads have been skilfully pressed into your man's anus, they are pulled out at the moment of his orgasm. This carefully timed bonus seriously increases his climatic sensation.

All sex toys need to be scrupulously cleaned before reuse, and don't use vaginal toys for anal sex. Clothing your sex toys in condoms reduces the risk of sexually transmitted diseases.

Anal plugs are often used by men and women who want anal stimulation during masturbation or intercourse. Plugs come in a variety of sizes and materials.

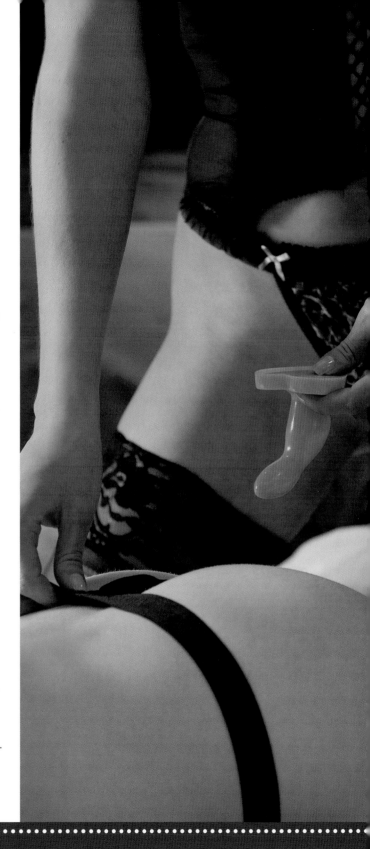

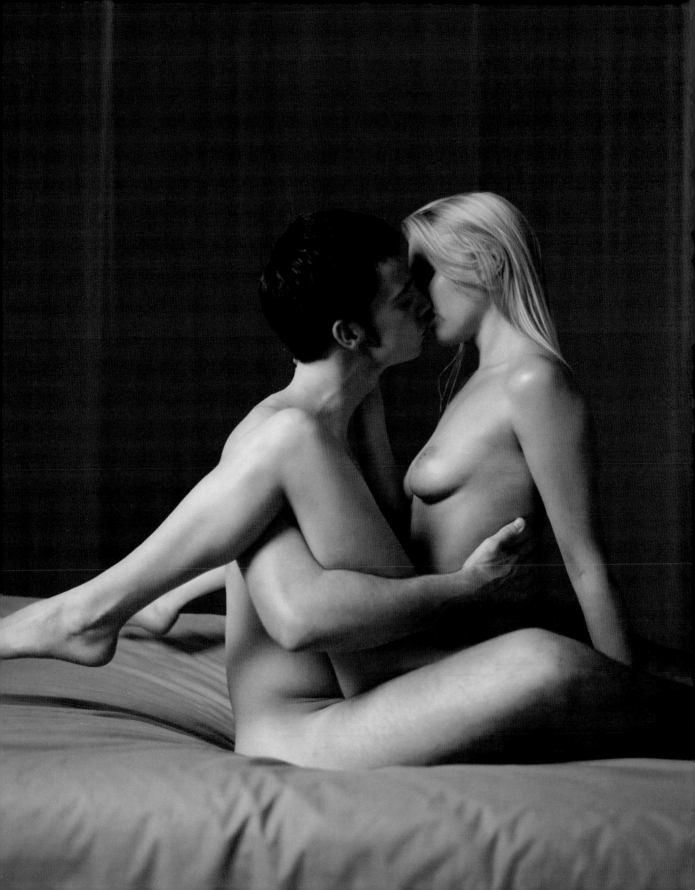

dominatrix

This teasing position is all hers, as she climbs over him to satisfy her desires. It usually works best when performed by a strong man and a light woman.

As he sits on the bed, she climbs on top of him, resting her legs over his arms and moving from side to side. This is a surprisingly arousing stroke for her as it puts pressure on a number of sensitive spots on the outer entrance of the vagina.

To add to their mutual pleasure, she can tease him by straddling him without allowing him to penetrate her immediately. Taunting him like this will lead to greater pleasure when they finally begin to make love.

Like most good things, truly erotic sex is something to be lingered over, taken slowly and deliberately, and thought about a great deal. If you're just getting to know someone, spinning out your time together without having intercourse can result in a very sexy build-up of excitement. If you are already lovers, postponing sex for a while can make your relationship feel like a new one again. The secret to playing "wait-for-it" games is to tease and arouse your lover without letting him or her know what you're doing.

On the emotional side, these games build up the thrill of sexuality in your brain. Because sexual fulfilment is delayed it becomes the only thing on your mind, and the longer you force yourselves to wait, the more tantalized you both become. On the physical side, the build-up of sexual tension (resulting in muscular contractions in the sex organs) means that, when they finally arrive, your orgasms can be longer and stronger than those resulting from immediate gratification.

• SEXY GAMES TO PLAY

Here are suggestions for sexy games you and your partner might like to play, or use as a basis for your own imaginative inventions. Agree that you will do whatever activity your partner orders. Take turns (for example, on alternate nights) to do anything sexual and enjoyable with each other except for intercourse. Give your partner boundaries for their behavior and punish them if they move beyond them—one punishment might be light caning or spanking. The game is more fun if the boundaries are impossible to stick to. Try a bit of role-playing: pretend she's a shy, totally inexperienced virgin and he's a sophisticated seducer. Or pretend he is an inexperienced youth and she is a seductive, experienced older woman. The possibilities are endless.

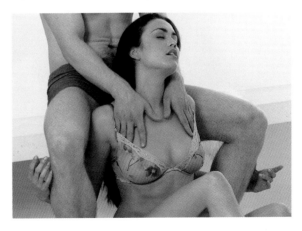

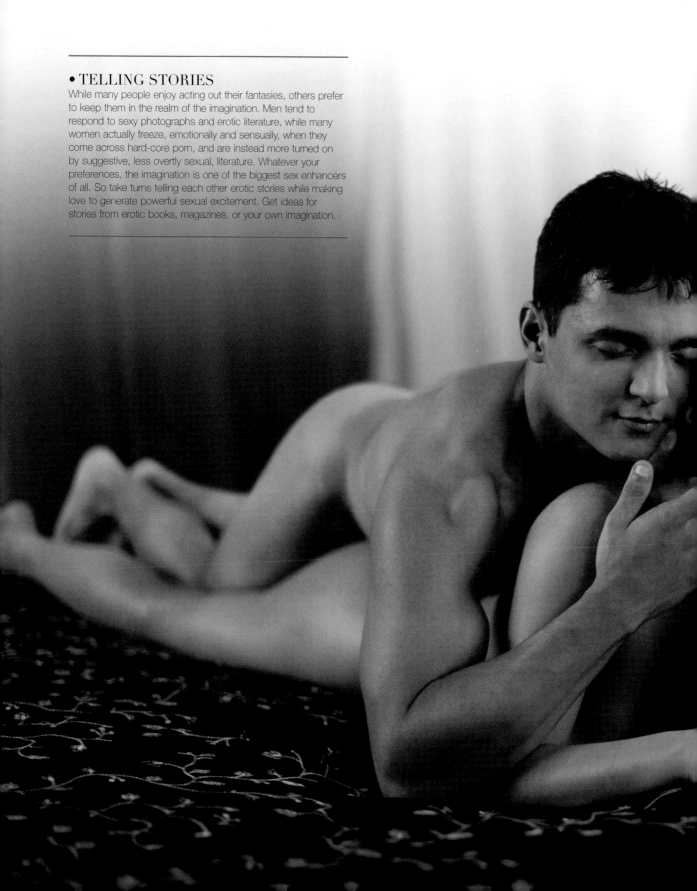

• TELLING STORIES

While many people enjoy acting out their fantasies, others prefer to keep them in the realm of the imagination. Men tend to respond to sexy photographs and erotic literature, while many women actually freeze, emotionally and sensually, when they come across hard-core porn, and are instead more turned on by suggestive, less overtly sexual, literature. Whatever your preferences, the imagination is one of the biggest sex enhancers of all. So take turns telling each other erotic stories while making love to generate powerful sexual excitement. Get ideas for stories from erotic books, magazines, or your own imagination.

legs together

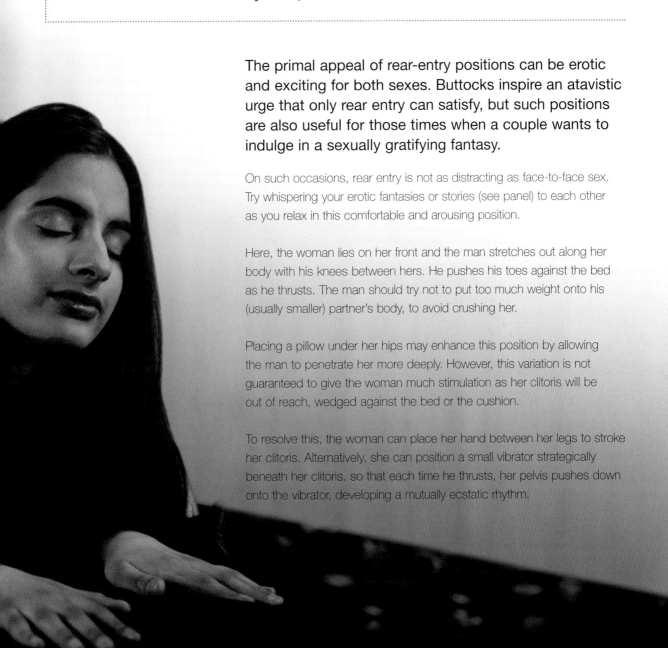

The primal appeal of rear-entry positions can be erotic and exciting for both sexes. Buttocks inspire an atavistic urge that only rear entry can satisfy, but such positions are also useful for those times when a couple wants to indulge in a sexually gratifying fantasy.

On such occasions, rear entry is not as distracting as face-to-face sex. Try whispering your erotic fantasies or stories (see panel) to each other as you relax in this comfortable and arousing position.

Here, the woman lies on her front and the man stretches out along her body with his knees between hers. He pushes his toes against the bed as he thrusts. The man should try not to put too much weight onto his (usually smaller) partner's body, to avoid crushing her.

Placing a pillow under her hips may enhance this position by allowing the man to penetrate her more deeply. However, this variation is not guaranteed to give the woman much stimulation as her clitoris will be out of reach, wedged against the bed or the cushion.

To resolve this, the woman can place her hand between her legs to stroke her clitoris. Alternatively, she can position a small vibrator strategically beneath her clitoris, so that each time he thrusts, her pelvis pushes down onto the vibrator, developing a mutually ecstatic rhythm.

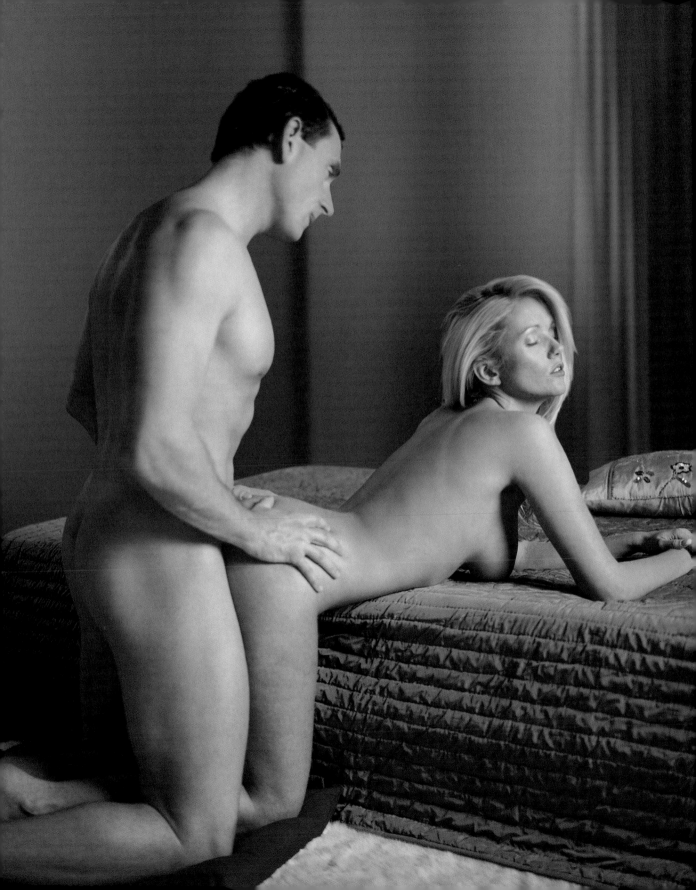

the quickie

Spontaneous sex features regularly in our lives in this busy era. But that doesn't mean it has to be inferior to more languid session. Just the idea of a stolen quickie can be extremely erotic.

In this rear-entry position, the woman lies face down across a bed with her knees on the floor, or stands, and leans forward over the bed. This is a profoundly tantalizing position, whether she is clothed or naked, offering immediate access even for just a few precious moments. From here, the man is able to thrust freely, while she is supported by the bed and can enjoy his vigorous attentions. She may be excited by deep penetration, and the man can give her extra thrills by caressing her clitoris with his hands.

This position is easy to get out of should you be interrupted unexpectedly, so you can try it whenever the mood takes you: before work, as a prelude to dinner, or even if the kids are expected any moment.

Seducing your lover for a quickie shows them how irresistible you find them, and it encourages you to have sex even when you think you don't have time.

Unexpected seductions can happen anywhere, at any time. Greet your lover at the door wearing skimpy underwear or just a smile; wait for them outside the bathroom door with a kiss, then remove their towel;

distract them from the TV, computer, or household chores by kissing their neck, or simply strip off and see what happens next. It's worth remembering that quick sex is better than no sex at all, and snatching time together can immediately boost your intimacy, your emotional bond, and your well-being.

• BATHROOM SEX

Sex in the bathroom is delightful in that it offers opportunities for both quick and urgent satisfaction, and long, lingering pampering. If you find few opportunities for more extended lovemaking, try sharing a shower together in the morning: the combination of warm water and soapy skin may lend itself naturally to mutual masturbation, or intercourse in standing positions such as "hands down" (see page 153). Alternatively, lock yourselves away together for the evening and try a sensual bathing ritual. Soapy, slippery hands and fingers arouse physical sensations all over the skin, and the gradual "soaping" massage can encourage your lover to accept caresses that they wouldn't normally be comfortable with.

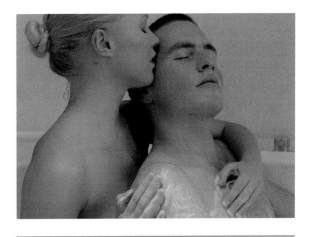

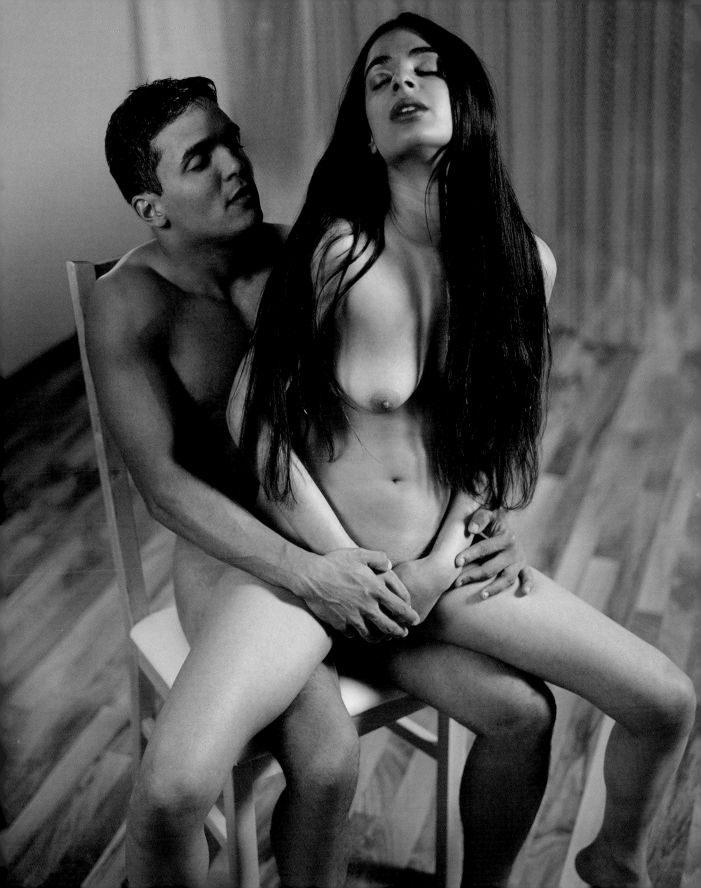

sitting pretty

Sit on his knee and feel his hands all over you

This is the sort of playful position that could develop from a couple casually fooling around together, as the woman sits on her man's knee, chatting or cuddling at the end of the day.

The man sits on a chair or the edge of the bed and the woman sits astride him with her back to him. She rests her feet on the floor so that she can gently rock backward and forward on his penis.

His movements are restricted, but his hands and lips are free to explore and pleasure his woman's body to the maximum. He can awaken her erotic senses with your hands, lips, tongue, and teeth. Each movement will heighten desire and anticipation.

Men: as you nibble and bite your way along your woman's body, you might choose to make a soft humming sound as you exhale. The vibrations will feel tantalizingly erotic to your woman. Try dainty nibbles, where the teeth just glide over the surface of her skin, to send quivers of pleasure down her spine, and alternate them with stronger, sucking bites that pull gently at a larger area of her skin.

To increase her pleasure, either partner can stimulate the woman's clitoris in this position with their fingers or a sex toy. The spontaneity of this intimate pose can add to the excitement you both feel.

To give your woman an added treat, enhance the sensations she receives from your stroking by strapping a vibrating massager to your hand. Or massage her with a scratchy bath mitt filled with oil. The oil will seep on to her skin so she experiences a delicious combination of rough and smooth.

•"YOU ARE MY SEXUAL SLAVE"

You might want to extend the possibilities for controlling your man in this position, or any similar male submissive pose. Blindfold him and tie him to a chair or bedpost. Tell him that he will now be your sexual slave and must be ready to obey every instruction. Try to convince him that there is another person in the room whom he must obey, and disguise your voice and change the way you walk and move to strengthen the illusion. Demand that he use sex toys on you (see pages 164–165), and reward him with strokes and kisses in his favorite places. Since your man cannot see who is performing the sexual acts on him, his imagination is free to run wild. Enjoy teasing and tormenting him before finally allowing him to penetrate you.

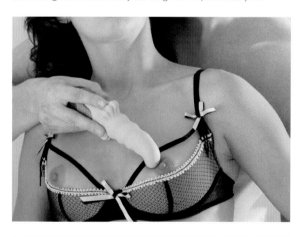

monkey moves

Sit on his lap and curl your limbs around him like a monkey

In this wonderfully intimate position, the woman climbs on her man, wraps her limbs around him, then teases him to a climax by gyrating on his penis.

In this position, the man plays the submissive role. He has little opportunity to move, but can enjoy the intimacy and emotional contact as she makes love to him. She can enjoy taking control, matching the speed and intensity of thrusting to her desires.

The man sits on the bed or floor with his legs out in front of him. His woman straddles him, curls her legs around his back, then leans back on her outstretched hand to lever her pelvis up and down, round and round in a steady thrusting motion.

• FLAUNT YOURSELF

Many women find it hard to act the exhibitionist in front of their man, and yet most men adore being a voyeur. Your partner may long to watch you perform a lap dance or a striptease, or masturbate, or be the ravisher or extravagantly sexual. Men are turned on far more than women by what they see, and one of the best ways to impress your man is to put on a show for him. Work out a striptease or sexy dance for him, or simply allow yourself to express your sexual feelings in front of him. Or ask him what sex act he would most like to see you perform.

The man can place his hand beneath her buttocks to support her as she moves, or simply to caress them. Many women find this action especially arousing. If she likes, he can also stretch her buttocks slightly to the side, allowing increased pressure on the perineum to generate exciting sensations.

Most men will enjoy the voyeuristic nature of this pose. He can watch her make love to him, while still being able to kiss, caress, and make sexy eye contact.

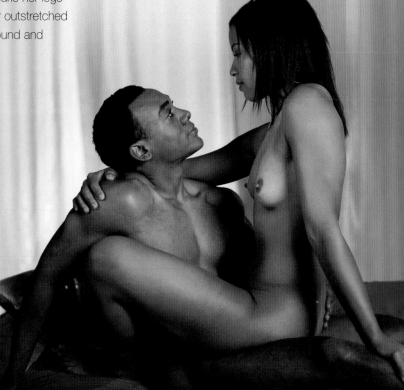

wash and brush up

Ravish your woman in the bathroom for impromptu ecstasy

Some of the most fantastic sex takes place while your and your partner are standing up. There is nothing quite like falling on each other in such a rush of passion that you just do it right now.

There are plenty of delicious upright positions to choose from wherever you are. You can use a number of different props to support you in upright sexual endeavors, such as a wall, or the stairs. A washbasin is often at the ideal height for upright sex, provided

that it is securely fixed to the wall or floor. And it often has the added thrill of a mirror fitted above, for the voyeuristic pleasure of watching yourselves.

The woman perches her bottom on the edge of the basin and grips his waist with her knees. He leans over her to penetrate. Both partners will need to hold on tightly to one another, but the angle of penetration mean that his penis can stimulate her clitoris, and both may find that the close thrusting brings them to an explosive climax—perfect for a quickie before work.

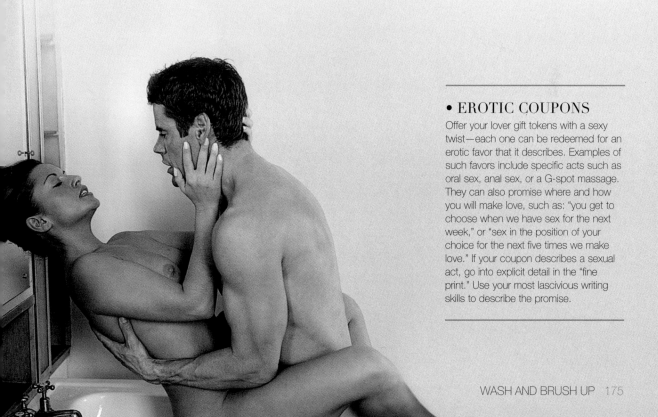

• EROTIC COUPONS

Offer your lover gift tokens with a sexy twist—each one can be redeemed for an erotic favor that it describes. Examples of such favors include specific acts such as oral sex, anal sex, or a G-spot massage. They can also promise where and how you will make love, such as: "you get to choose when we have sex for the next week," or "sex in the position of your choice for the next five times we make love." If your coupon describes a sexual act, go into explicit detail in the "fine print." Use your most lascivious writing skills to describe the promise.

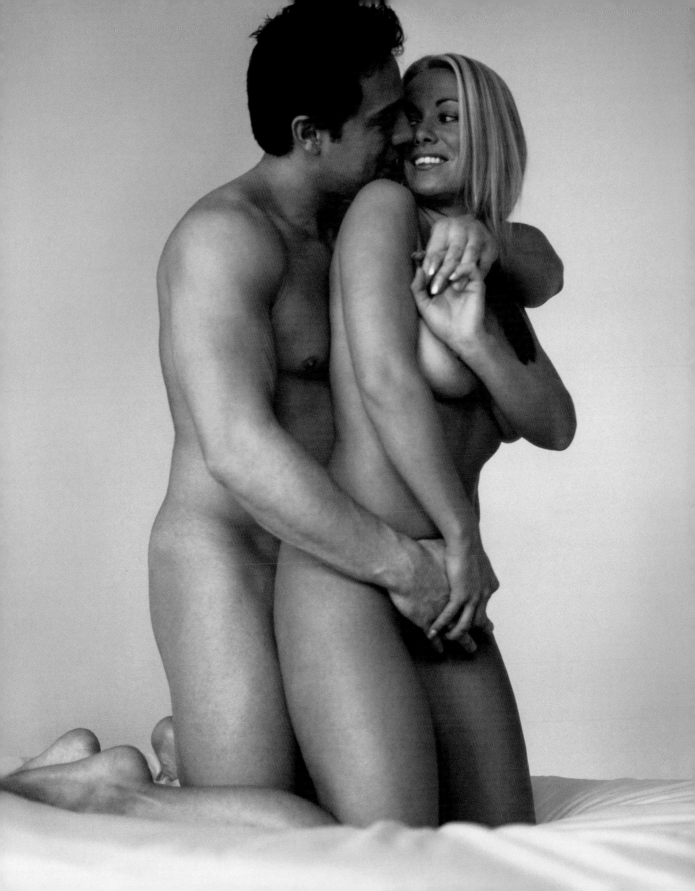

sensual feast

Caress and stroke your woman for sense-sational sex

This sexy kneeling position is wonderfully versatile as both partners have their hands free to stroke and caress each other, and it is easy to move into other rear-entry positions.

The woman kneels on the bed and her man kneels behind her to penetrate. Embracing, stroking, and kissing your partner while you're both upright feels wonderfully erotic. If she matches his thrusts and keeps her bottom close to his pelvis, the couple can move together with rhythmic intensity. Either partner can stimulate her clitoris with their fingers while thrusting, to make this position more exciting for her.

To heighten your excitement in this position, indulge in some sensuous stroking before you move on to lovemaking. Equip yourselves with squares of arousing fabrics such as silk or velvet. Kneel on the bed together, or on a large piece of velvet on the floor. Now stroke every inch of each others' skin with each of your sensual fabrics in turn.

You can whisk the materials across the body, use them to tickle, tease, and finally massage all your partner's hot spots—breasts, chest, neck, buttocks, and thighs. Avoid their genitals at first: the anticipation will serve to heighten your partner's excitement. Resist touching their most intimate areas until you have thoroughly pleasured the rest of their body.

When venturing into the world of exotic sex, among the first delights to incorporate into your love life are sensual props. The teasing of velvet or the slither of silk across your skin can produce exquisite sensations. Other sensual materials include fur, leather, PVC, or rough materials like canvas or an exfoliating mitt.

• BOX OF DELIGHTS

Prepare a box of sexual toys and tricks for your and your lover's delight. The ideal adult toy chest is discreet and attractive, such as a plain box, beautifully finished with black or red lacquer on the outside. The interior might be padded with gleaming satin or wispy chiffon. Inside you might want to keep souvenirs, such as a set of your lover's underwear, a goody bag containing handcuffs, self-adhesive tattoos, a blindfold, a slinky PVC or rubber outfit or underwear, a paddle, or a fur collar and leash. You could add a vibrator, massage oil, and erotic books or photographs. Since you won't want any curious passers-by to delve into the mysteries of your coffer uninvited, put a padlock on it. A beautiful silver or gold one will add to the intrigue.

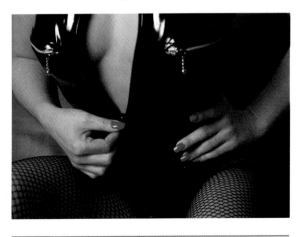

kneeling master

Dominate your woman to bring her intense pleasure

Many couples adore rear-entry kneeling positions because they lend themselves easily to games of light bondage, domination, and control.

In "kneeling master," the woman plays the submissive role by kneeling on all fours on the bed and resting her forearms and head on the bed. He enters from behind, and her lowered body is supported by the bed against her lover's vigorous thrusts.

In this position, she may find the submissive role is very restful, as she lets her partner take control of her body and the rhythmic thrusting of lovemaking. To gain more stimulation from this position, she can use her hands or a vibrator against her clitoris to

maximize the stimulation of her partner's thrusts. This leaves his hands free to roam across her back and breasts, which can be erotic for both partners.

Because the woman supports herself in this position, the man does not have to hold his body weight off his partner in the same way as for other rear-entry positions. This allows him to enjoy the position at a leisurely pace, without muscular exertion.

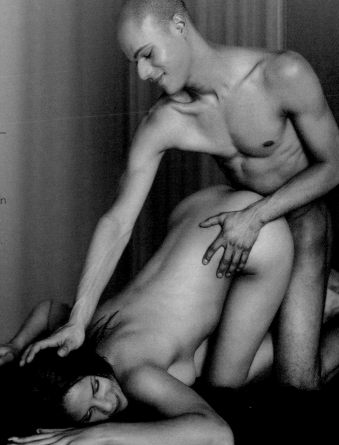

• EROTIC GIFTS

Don't forget to combine experiments in sexual domination with moments of tenderness. A sexy surprise present at any time of year is a great way to make your lover feel desired. Be creative in the way that you offer your gifts; for example, try exotic fruit that is just waiting to be eaten directly from your body, or a bunch of red roses (thornless ones) to use as an innovative spanking tool. Or you could leave your partner an extra-special present under their pillow, such as a penis-head stimulator for him, a fingertip vibrator for her, or a toy duck that vibrates for both of you to enjoy in the bath.

animal attraction

Let out your inner animal and abandon yourselves to pleasure

Many ancient sex manuals sought inspiration from the mating habits of animals, such as elephants or tigers. By giving into these animalistic urges, lovers can extend their sexual repertoire.

In this position, inspired by the mating techniques of elephants, the woman lies on her front and the man supports himself on his arms, entering her powerfully from the rear. The man can rear up from his woman with the small of his back arched inward as he thrusts deeply into her from this position.

The sensations of taking and being taken can be thrilling for both partners. The primitive power this affords can greatly add to his excitement and lend your lovemaking a special eroticism. Men: feel free to give vent to a primeval yell.

This may be not the sexiest of lovemaking positions for her, since her clitoris receives little stimulation. The very idea of this pose, however, can prove to be highly seductive. By pressing her thighs together, she can increase the sexual friction between his penis and her vagina, to improve sensation for both.

• EROTIC RECORDINGS

Apart from stocking up on what you consider to be really sexy music, it's worth thinking about making your own recordings. You can record all kinds of sexy blandishments to excite your partner when you aren't together. You might record some erotic short stories, your own sounds of lovemaking, an endless list of sexual praise, or conversations or commands in two voices, so that your partner is able to fantasize about the presence of two of you in the room. Everything is subjective, and what one person thinks is erotic may not be for another, so couples will need to experiment to find the sounds that turn each other on, and heighten their anticipation for the real thing.

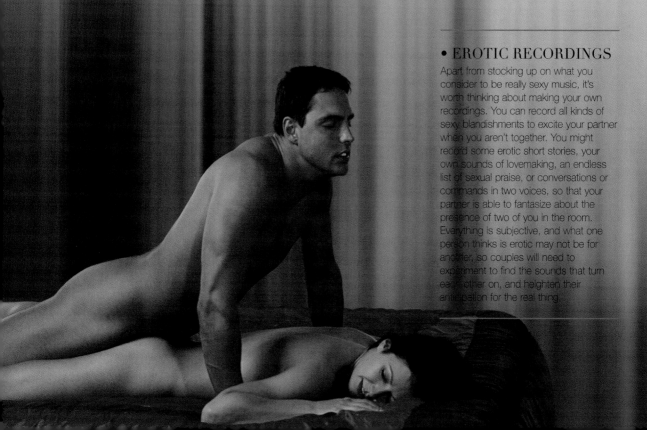

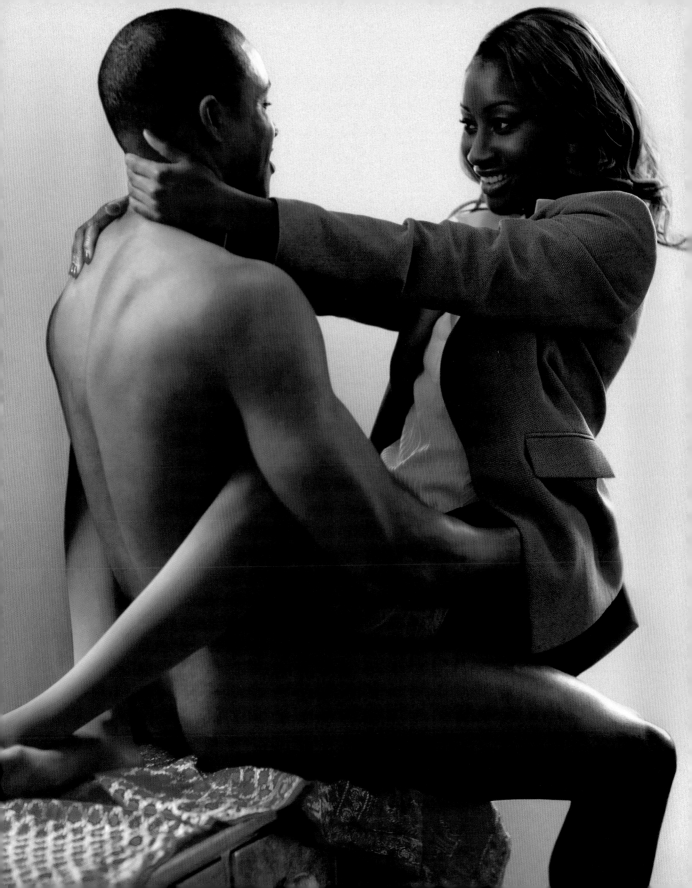

sudden seduction

One of the great killers of good sex is boredom. However much you adore your partner, if you have made love in the same way for years, then sex just won't be as erotic as it used to be.

The good news is that only one of you has to change one item in that fixed pattern, such as what you wear, your sexual position or where you make love, and sex takes on a new lease of life. The secret is to keep an open mind about trying new things, and be unafraid to make some slightly different moves.

Sex in the sitting position is ideal for an impromptu session when time is short, or you want to spring a surprise seduction on your lover. Its eroticism lies in the novelty value, and the fact that the woman doesn't need to remove her clothes so it feels spontaneous.

Here, the man sits on the edge of the bed or sofa, with his feet on the floor. The woman sits on his lap, then wraps her arms round his neck and her legs round his back to allow him to penetrate her deeply. The couple can then move as they please. By rocking backward and forward on his penis, she can give him orgasmic strokes bound to please him.

If you are looking for changes in your sex life, one of the easiest is the way you dress. If you always make love naked, then one of you could choose to wear a special costume for extra excitement.

When dressing for sex, the rules are simple: wear tight clothes that emphasize the curves and contours of the body and draw the eye to the breasts, chest, legs, buttocks, or genitals. Clothes should be difficult for your partner to take off, to tantalize them further, but easy for you to slip out of at the right moment.

• EROTIC DRESSING

Wearing something unexpected to shock your partner can be a source of erotic power. To spice up your sex life, try subverting your normal dress codes. For example, if you normally dress down in your everyday life, try dressing up for sex. If you tend to wear conservative clothes, dress provocatively for a change. Devote a special part of your wardrobe to sex games. If you're a woman who usually wears pale cosmetics, try experimenting with deep crimson lipstick: huge dark lips are often seen as sensual. Eye shadow on a man can also be attractive to some women. And because underwear is the last item of clothing that you shed before sex, it has an important symbolic value. When it is silky, lacy, or made of PVC, it can have a wonderfully sensual effect.

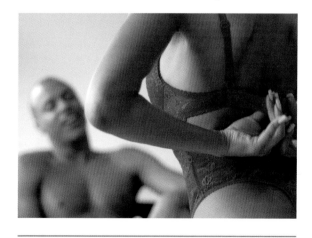

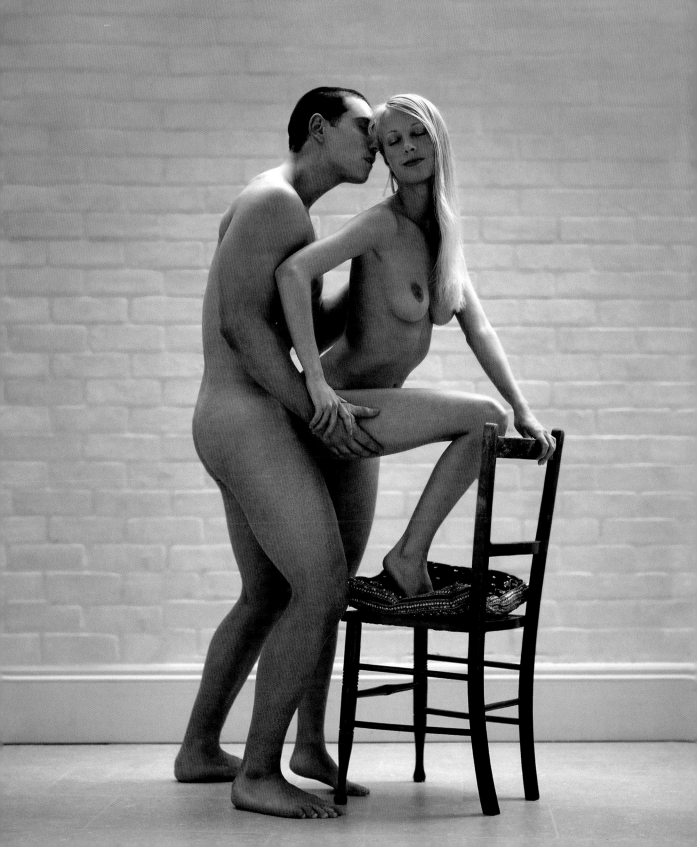

a leg lifted

Slide her leg onto a chair and begin your own private fantasy

Human beings are artistic as well as inventive. By using props such as chairs or washbasins, couples can get themselves into wonderfully sensual positions, and create erotic stories too.

For him, this position allows for deep penetration and enables him to control the depth and the power of his thrusts for maximum stimulation. He can begin by moving slowly, teasing her, then hold her around the waist to pull her deeper onto his penis.

Women will also find this position rewarding. As the man thrusts he can move his fingers round to stroke her clitoris in rhythm, or she can touch herself if she wants to. The action of his hips pounding against her buttocks, and his penis sliding across her perineum, can prove highly arousing.

Couples can make this position as raunchy or as tender as they choose, by turning to kiss one another, or whispering dirty thoughts in each others' ears. Why might she be asked to raise her leg as he slips into her from the rear? Let your imaginations run wild.

You could also use a mirror to add excitement. Seeing yourself and your partner in this imaginative sexual position can be highly arousing. Or you could pretend that the mirror is a window into another room, where two lovers are performing especially for you.

You could angle the mirror to watch his penis moving in and out, so that the reflection becomes a kind of porn movie in which you both get to star. Or one of you might order the other to do something sexual that they may never have seen themselves doing before.

• NAUGHTY GAMES

Naughty games are so-called because they explore the darker side of sex, otherwise known as "BDSM." This stands for "bondage, domination, submission, and masochism." Choose your role as either "dom" or "sub." As the dom you must dress powerfully. If you are the sub, all you need are a few leather straps or chains strategically placed. Now act out one of these scenarios. You are a dungeon master/mistress and your lover is your victim. You own a grand house and your lover is your servant. You are a professor and your lover is an errant student. You are are the prison warden and your lover is the prisoner. The aim is for the dom to punish the sub by, for example, inflicting mild discomfort or humiliation, restraining movement, or giving and then withdrawing sexual stimulation.

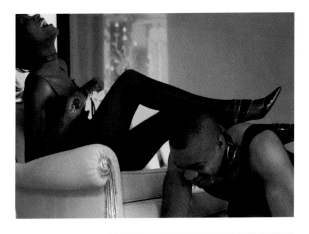

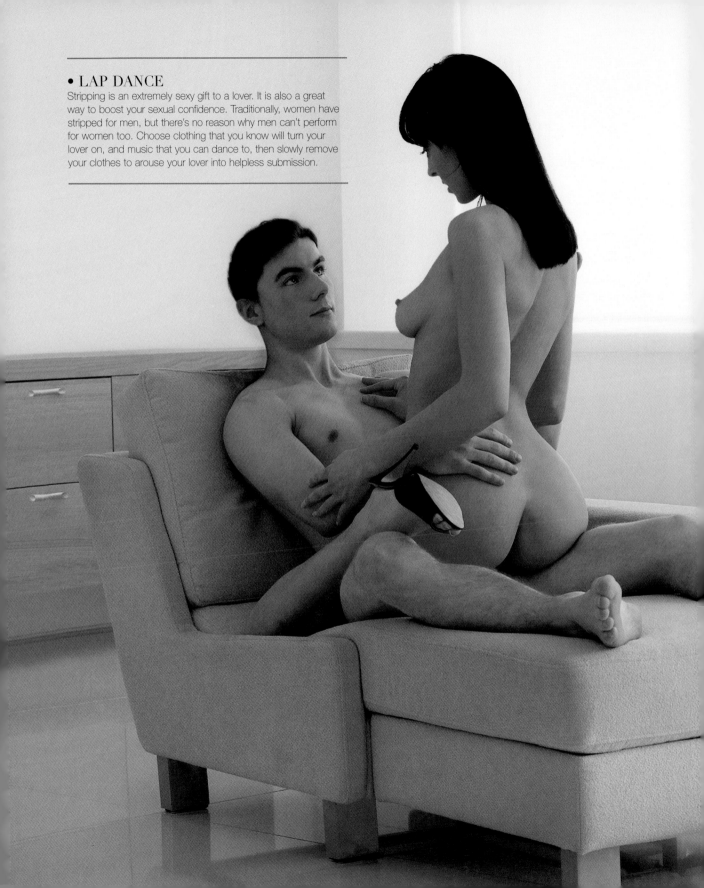

• LAP DANCE

Stripping is an extremely sexy gift to a lover. It is also a great way to boost your sexual confidence. Traditionally, women have stripped for men, but there's no reason why men can't perform for women too. Choose clothing that you know will turn your lover on, and music that you can dance to, then slowly remove your clothes to arouse your lover into helpless submission.

heel power

Strip down to your shoes, then seduce him any way you like it

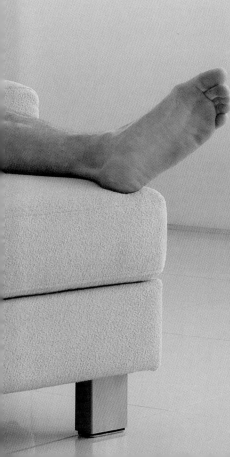

Take a tip from the porn stars and beg, borrow, or steal a pair of hooker-style high heels. They will boost your confidence as well as your height. Lap and pole dancers wear them for their sexy, glamorous appearance, and because they give a trademark hip-sway as you walk.

This position is perfect for pouncing on your man, perhaps when he's watching TV or relaxing in bed. The woman straddles him and sits down on him. Once he's penetrated her, she has the freedom to thrust or move up and down to find the angle that gives her most stimulation.

If she wants to draw out the seduction prior to sex, she can play her role to the maximum by standing with one foot on a chair, sexily unrolling her stockings, or playfully resting her heel on his thigh, crotch, or chest. Or she can make it part of a role-play and pretend that she is a pole dancer auditioning for a job in front of the demanding owner of an exotic dancing club. She's desperate for the job, so she is prepared to do almost anything—but not without teasing him along the way.

She can tease him into helpless desire by promising sex, but then withholding it at the very last minute, drawing away as from him even as she allows the head of his penis to slip inside her. Women-on-top positions are ideally suited to games like this. Women: keep your heels on during sex—even if everything else comes off.

The tempo of sex gathers new shape when the woman takes charge. Not only can she ensure that she is stimulated in all the important areas, but the lovemaking takes on new excitement for her man as well.

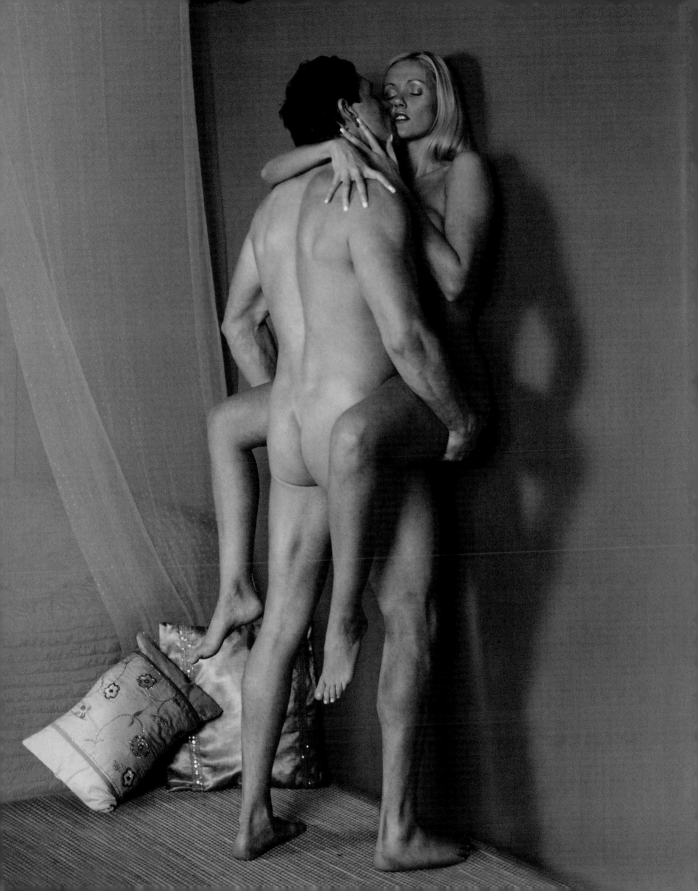

against a wall

Press her to the wall and let her feel how much you want her

Standing sex celebrates irrepressible lust and desire. There is a place in everyone's sex life for erotic immediacy. Show the strength of your attraction to each other by being impulsive and abandoned.

When passion suddenly overwhelms us, lovers may desire spontaneous sex standing in the nearest available private space. This position is ideal for making love in a cubicle, against a wall, a tree, or leaning into one another.

The woman wraps her legs as tightly as possible around the man's waist, holds onto his shoulders, and keeps her back straight against the wall. If he is strong, the man can thrust satisfactorily while lifting his partner at the same time, and because she is supported by the wall and he is braced against her, he can thrust freely and passionately.

At this height and angle, her clitoris is stretched and exposed and, therefore, more likely to be affected by the thrust and pull of intercourse. She should lift her thighs up higher against her man's to achieve greater penetration as he thrusts. This will enhance his enjoyment, and increase her stimulation.

This can be an outrageously exciting position, particularly if you are outside the house and there is the danger of getting caught. The risk of discovery can heighten sexual arousal, as adrenaline adds a natural chemical zap to the proceedings. Some people, however, get so anxious about being caught in the act that they find it hard to get aroused. A safer, but still exciting, option might be to wait for the neighbors to go out, and then try this one in the privacy of your yard or terrace.

• SEX ANYWHERE, ANY TIME

If you live in a town or a city, novel locations for sex include car parks, stairwells, elevators, and offices. You need to be adept at spotting opportunities for privacy if you want to enjoy quickie, stand-up sex. Men: dress for the occasion by leaving your underwear at home. Women: wear a skirt or dress. One sex trick is to have part-private, part-public sex by keeping your clothes on and leaning out of a window—this works best if you're high up, say in a hotel room looking down on a busy street. He enters her from behind and keeps his movements small and barely discernible. It's vital, however, to make love where you can't be seen or you'll be in trouble with the authorities. One simple, sexy option is just to enjoy the luxury of a hotel bedroom.

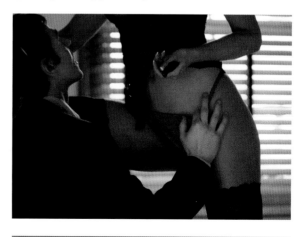

index

A

acrobatic ecstasy 8, 100–41

anal intercourse 158–9

anal plug (butt plug) 164, 165

anal stimulation 164

    hers 87, 94, 158, 159

    his 157, 165

angles of penetration 17, 20, 23, 34, 53, 75, 77, 80, 87, 93, 95

animal attraction/power 33, 179

ankle hold 109

arch, lovers' 129

arching back 134

arms outstretched 26

arousal 65, 96, 129

    nine levels of 129

    signs 23

B

bareback rider 118

baths and showers 97, 137, 139, 171, 174

bed and bedroom

    beyond the 136–7, 139

    day in the 90

Beautrais maneuver 74

belly-to-belly 53

biting and nibbling 27, 39, 173

blindfolds 151, 164, 173, 177

bondage and restraints 149, 151, 152, 173

    thoughts of 152

bottom, spanking see spanking

bottoms up 141

breast

    he kissing hers 26

    he stroking/touching hers 15

    she stroking/touching herself 15

    see also nipples

butt (anal) plugs 164, 165

buttock see bottoms up; caning; spanking

C

caning 150, 167

cat, the 97

chairs 134, 137, 140, 159, 163, 183, 185

chakras 130

chest, stroking 70

circling exercise 118

circling strokes 42–3, 70

climax see orgasm

clitoral stimulation 15, 17, 19, 23, 33, 34, 46, 47, 63, 65, 72, 87, 99, 103, 104, 105, 113, 115, 119, 123, 133, 135, 139, 175, 187

    manual, by herself 34, 81, 92, 93, 97, 112, 125, 169, 173, 177, 178, 183

    manual, by him 19, 32, 33, 35, 37, 71, 79, 93, 96, 107, 117,147, 152, 155, 159, 171, 173, 177, 183

    oral stimulation 82, 83

    rear-entry position 33

    vibrators see vibrators

closeness, maximum/extreme 15, 17, 22, 32, 98

clothes see cross-dressing; dressing-up; stripping

condoms 51, 165

    anal sex 158, 159

cross-dressing and drag

    for her 161

    for him 155

cross-legged 59, 93, 112

crush, sexy 17

cunnilingus 82, 83

curling up 32

cushions and pillows 16, 20, 34, 49, 50, 120, 155, 162, 169

D

day in bed 90

deep penetration 17, 21, 23, 31, 33, 34, 39, 50, 51, 57, 63, 77, 103, 115, 118, 119, 120, 121, 124, 133, 149, 159, 161, 169, 171, 179, 181, 183

    Tao sets of nine 58

    see also thrusting

deep yawn 57

deer exercise

    for men 111

    for women 111

desire 65

    love's, 125

divinely deep 113

dominance see punishment/reward games; submission and dominance

drag see cross-dressing

dressing-up 181

    see also cross-dressing; stripping

E

easy love 46

embraces, erotic 6, 10–53

encircling 59

entwining of legs see legs

erectile dysfunction 62, 93

erogenous zones 27, 81, 125, 126, 158

exercises see Pilates; strengthening exercises; yoga

exhibitionism 140, 174

his 70, 115
"nothing" session 76
novelty 9, 29, 129, 136, 137, 163, 181
nurse and patient 150, 183

O

odor, body 73
oil wrestling 51
on-top positions
    man 13–21, 34, 57, 62, 75, 123,
      131, 146
    woman 22, 28–9, 38, 49, 65,
      87–91, 93–5, 99, 116, 117,
      132, 134–5, 152, 155,
      161–2, 167, 185
oral stimulation 82–5
orgasm/climax (either partner) 65, 67,
    93, 107, 121
    whole-body 61
orgasm/climax (hers) 14
    delaying 77
    G-spot 68, 77
    multiple 99
orgasm/climax (his) 32
    delaying 36, 74, 79, 95, 121
    multiple 153
ostrich, tail of the 111
outdoor sex 136, 137, 139

P

P-spot 156, 165
paddle sensuous, 76
pelvic floor exercises see strengthening
    exercise
penis
    angles of penetration 17, 20, 23,
      53, 75, 77, 80, 87, 93, 95
    deep penetration see deep
      penetration
    erectile dysfunction 62, 93

exercise 120
frenulum 20, 82, 120
friction between vagina and 28, 32,
    37, 46, 67, 72, 96, 119, 121,
    123, 179
oral stimulation 82
stimulation by her 31, 69, 71,
    108, 120
stimulation by himself 66
thrusting motions 104, 133,
    178
perineum, hers 22, 83, 96
perineum, his 16, 49
    Jen Mo point 79
pheromones 29
phone sex 57, 136
piercing embrace 133
Pilates 102
pillows and cushions 16, 20, 34, 49,
    50, 120, 155, 162, 169
playful pleasure 119
press, the 73
pressed thighs 67, 81, 96
pressing together 121
pressure, steady 72
professor and student 150, 183
props 9, 141, 163, 164, 175,
    177, 183
prostate (P) spot 156, 165
prostitute (hooker) and client 183
punishment/reward games 139, 145,
    150, 167, 183
pupil and teacher 150, 183
puppy love, 35

Q R

quick–quick–slow rhythm 87, 132
quickie, the 171, 175, 187
racing horse 149
raised legs 17, 23, 57, 67, 68, 76, 93,

    96, 107, 109, 111, 124, 125
rear-entry sex 25, 32, 34–7, 41, 49, 72,
    97, 116, 147, 153, 169, 171,
    177–9, 187
recording 179
repose, woman in 99
resting 32
restraints see bondage
reward/punishment 139, 145, 150, 167,
    183
rocking horse 65
role play 150–1
reversal (of power) 152, 155, 161
    submission and dominance see
      punishment/reward; submission
      and dominance

S

scissors 75
see-saw 146
"seizure" technique 72
self (woman)
    clitoral stimulation 34, 81, 92, 93,
      97, 112, 125, 169, 173, 177,
      178, 183
    stroking,15, 35
sensation, maximum 8, 45–99
    see also skin; strokes
sets of nine, Taoist 58, 132
sex games and fantasies 8, 112, 142–87
sex toys 164–5, 177
    inventor fantasy 152
    male 156
    vibrators see vibrators
sexual mapping 61
sexual response, 65
sexual variety 6, 9, 107, 136, 163, 181
shake, sensational 124
shoes 11, 185
shoulder blade (her) sensitive spot, 121

Acknowledgments

DK would like to thank Steve Crozier and MDP for retouching, Sharon Amos for proofreading, Laura Mingozzi for design assistance, and Laurence Errington for indexing.

Please note:

It is assumed that couples are monogamous and have been tested for sexually transmitted infections. Always practise safe and responsible sex, and consult a doctor if you have a condition that might preclude strenuous sexual activity. Challenging intercourse positions might put a strain on your back or other body parts—do not attempt them if you have injuries or ailments and consult your doctor for advice beforehand if you are concerned. Sex in public places should only be undertaken with due consideration of the law and the sensibilities of others. The author and publisher do not accept any responsibility for any injury or ailment caused by following any of the suggestions contained in this book.